Psychoanalysis as a Science

Psychoanalysis as a Science

LEOPOLD BELLAK, M.D.
Emeritus Professor of Psychiatry
Albert Einstein College of Medicine/
Montefiore Medical Center
and
Clinical Professor of Psychology
Postdoctoral Program in Psychotherapy
New York University

With the Collaboration of

JAMES WALKUP, Ph.D.

ALLYN AND BACON
Boston   London   Toronto   Sydney   Tokyo   Singapore

Copyright © 1993 by Allyn and Bacon
A Division of Simon & Schuster, Inc.
160 Gould Street
Needham Heights, Massachusetts 02194

All rights reserved. No part of the material protected by this copyright notice may be reproduced or utilized in any form or by any means, electronic or mechanical, including photocopying, recording, or by any information storage and retrieval system, without written permission from the copyright owner.

Library of Congress Cataloging-in-Publication Data

Bellak, Leopold.
    Psychoanalysis as a science / Leopold Bellak ; with the collaboration of James Walkup.
      p.   cm.
    Includes bibliographical references and index.
    ISBN 0-205-13904-3
    1. Psychoanalysis. I. Walkup, James. II. Title.
    [DNLM: 1. Psychoanalysis. 2. Psychoanalytic Theory.
WM 460 B435p]
BF173.B39   1993
150.19'5—dc20
DNLM/DLC
for Library of Congress   92-10471
                                                                              CIP

Printed in the United States of America
10 9 8 7 6 5 4 3 2 1   96 95 94 93 92

*To W. Ernest Freud,
for a lifetime of loyal friendship*

Contents

Preface   *xi*

Chapter One • Methodology   *1*
   Introduction   1
   Some Basic Principles   3
   An Imaginary Operationalization   6
   Example One: Ego Assessment   9
   Example Two: Psychotherapy   11
   Methodology and the Mundane   13

Chapter Two • Psychoanalytic Theory of Personality as Learning Theory   *15*
   Introduction   15
   Oedipus Simplified   18
   Perceptual Learning   21

Chapter Three • Psychoanalysis as a Perceptual Theory   *25*
   Introduction   25
   Perception and Apperception   26
   Forms of Apperceptive Distortion   27
   A Restatement of the Metapsychology of Projecting:
      Apperceiving as a Variant of Perception   36
   Perception and Clinical Phenomena   40

viii   Contents

Chapter Four • *Psychoanalysis as a Trait Psychology*   47

Introduction   47
Traits   49
Psychoanalysis and Traits   50
Libidinal Development   51
Ego, Id, and Superego   57
Psychoanalytic Theory: "Types" and "Traits"   64
The Future   66

Chapter Five • *Psychoanalysis as Developmental Theory*   67

Introduction   67
Current Status   69
Freud's Early Sightings of Development   69
Freud on Developmental Theory   72
The Next Generation: Anna Freud
 and Melanie Klein   75
John Bowlby   78
Margaret Mahler   83
The Contemporary Scene   86
Dan Stern   87

Chapter Six • *An Operational Definition of the Ego*   95

Introduction   95
Freud and Ego Psychology   96
Ego Functions: A Brief History
 and Introduction   97
Rating Ego Functions   101
The Research Project   104
Ego Function Assessment and Therapeutic
 Response   105
The Broad Scope of Ego Function
 Assessment   108

Chapter Seven • *Philosophy and Psychoanalysis* 111

    Bad Feelings and Suspicion   111
    Ludwig Wittgenstein   112
    Causes, Reasons, and Little Red Books   115
    Text Appeal—Appealing to the Text   120
    Karl Popper   123
    Falsification and Standards of Science   124
    A Matter of Attitude   127

Chapter Eight • *Psychoanalysis as a Form of Treatment and a Subject of Research* 129

    Introduction to Research in Psychoanalysis   133
    What Makes Psychotherapy Researchable?   136
    A Brief Historical Background   137
    A Few Words for the Consumer   143
    Methods   144
    An Early Effort   148
    Some Contemporary Examples   151
    Conclusion: The Future   163

***Epilogue*   165**

***Bibliography*   171**

***Name Index*   181**

***Subject Index*   184**

Preface

Sigmund Freud's great contribution was to establish continuity between childhood and adult life, between waking thought and sleeping thought, and between "normal" behavior and pathological behavior. He introduced causality into psychological science; indeed, Freud *made* psychology a science. It is likely that psychoanalysis as a science will last for a long time to come, all its "doomsday-sayers" to the contrary.

I propose to demonstrate that most of Freud's hypotheses can be stated operationally and, in principle, can be experimentally verified, modified, or rejected. These hypotheses, arrived at piecemeal from clinical observation, permit one to perform the basic operations of science: to predict and to postdict (as G. W. Allport called it), and to make collateral inferences.

Freud inferred causality by finding a continuity between the symptoms of his patients and their childhood history. He found that when he could establish continuity where there was apparent discontinuity—a sudden onset of a symptom such as a paralyzed arm—the symptomatology made sense, without the patient being aware of the meaning. Thus Freud invented the unconscious as a construct (Bellak, 1959a, 1959b).

The world reacted to this construct as if it were a dire insult. Charles Darwin's doctrine of evolution—still embattled in some parts of this country—was hard enough to swallow. To think that man was not God's crowning creation but merely the result of adaptation was a heavy blow indeed. Galileo too had offended mankind before, by insisting that the earth was not the center of the universe. Such a heretical way of thinking endangered his life.

Freud now added further insult to injury. By implication, the construct of the unconscious affected the idea of free will. If we are merely the end product of our experience, and often are not even aware of what motivates us, where does free will fit in?

The church certainly did not take to these ideas. If there is no free will, what happens to the belief in sin? If one could act without being aware of the motivation—as eventually formulated in the insanity defense of some criminals—the whole world would be turned topsy-turvy. Needless to say, Freud was not a popular man in clerical circles.

In understanding Freud's explanation of the manifest discontinuity in his patients' lives, bear in mind that Freud was a child of the nineteenth century, of Helmholtz and the laws of thermodynamics and hydraulics. Boltzman was teaching only a few blocks away and Ernst Mach lived and worked even closer. With such influences, it is easy to understand how Freud came up with the idea that the offending memory was suppressed—as if by a hydraulic pump. Thus was born the concept of repression, with the evil spirits trying always to escape, like a steaming goulash in a pot with the lid clamped firmly down.

As we will see later, concepts like selective scanning and concepts of Gestalt psychology may do a much better job in our time to explain the phenomena of repression and discontinuity. The sophistication of the model has potential bearing on the interpretation of the clinical facts.

Psychoanalysis as a *theory of personality,* as a *theory of psychopathology,* and as a *theory and method of psychotherapy* suffers from terrible shortcomings. As an originator, Freud was carried away by the excitement of new insights and often went on to formulate new hypotheses without paying sufficient attention to how they fit in with earlier formulations. Also, Freud was surrounded by enthusiastic disciples who were not acquainted with even the rudiments of methodology then available. Then (and now) psychoanalysts were mostly physicians, who also had not learned anything about concept formation, methodology, statistics, and experimental design and procedure. The end result of these factors is a regrettable mire of valuable observations, useful working hypotheses, heuristic hunches from anecdotal material, flights of fancy, and a vocabulary that confuses more than it clarifies.

Alas, there is more evidence that Freud was human and that, among other things, his thought was influenced by his cultural milieu. This demonstrates itself quite clearly in the changes that psychoanalytic theory underwent in its process of transplantation from Vienna specifically, and Europe generally, when analysts fled from the Nazi holocaust to the United States. One of the central concepts of psychoanalysis as a therapy was (and is) the concept of transference, the idea that the patient "transfers" his feelings from past figures to the analyst. In the Viennese setting, there was the patient, suffering from all kinds of foibles; behind him sat the "Herr Professor," a *tabula rasa* and cool observer. In that capacity, he also served as a screen on which the patient projected all of his distortions. The therapeutic process was solely predicated upon the analysis of these distortions and resistances.

Then, in the 1940s, Franz Alexander, a Hungarian psychoanalyst transplanted to Chicago, came up with the idea that the persona of the analyst played an important role in the changes taking place in a patient: the patient underwent "a corrective emotional experience." That is, if for instance he suffered from his unconscious representation of a critical father, the presence of a benign and nonjudgmental Alexander would modify the internal imagery. Although this viewpoint is still disputed by the mainstream classical analysts, the interactionist view of the "countertransference" is widespread in the U.S. culture. It is quite acceptable that the analyst also participates as a human being, complete with love, rage, fear, and other emotions. These emotions must not only be acknowledged but are in themselves another useful guide to the analytic process.

There were other variables of the cultural milieu that

influenced the body of hypotheses of psychoanalysis, and came under criticism in the United States. Outstanding among these were some conceptions of the female psyche. In Freud's discussion of the psychological development of the little girl, she emerged as a less important version of the male for not having a penis. Of course male chauvinism was an ingrained part of European culture, but Freud's own knowledge of women, especially in the Biblical sense, was very limited. There is virtually no knowledge of Freud's having any interest in women prior to his involvement with his future wife. Because of his poor financial status and his inability to support a wife and children, they remained engaged for many years. Since the future Mrs. Freud lived in Hamburg and Sigmund lived in Vienna, and this was not the era of commercial air travel, the couple saw each other infrequently. There is also no indication that he ever dated anyone else during that period. The best guess historians have come up with is that Lou Andreas Salome tried valiantly to seduce him, but there was no suggestion that she succeeded as she did with Nietzsche and Mahler, among others. Finally, according to his biographer, Ernest Jones, in his forties Freud gave up intercourse entirely, saying that he was too old for it.

Helene Deutsch, one of Freud's closest disciples, was probably the first one to take critical exception to some of Freud's notions of the psychology of women. While she may have been developing some of these ideas in Vienna, they matured in Boston where she published her two-volume work on the psychology of women. While she remained a mainstream psychoanalyst, others like Karen Horney and Clara Thompson developed rigorous feminine psychoanalytic conceptions that led them to establish their own schools of thought.

It would be a profound pity, however, to let these artifacts of history camouflage the fact that many psychoanalytic hypotheses are experimentally verifiable, publicly demonstrable, and repeatable.

Experimentally controlled research could be directed toward examining the validity of an isolated concept, such as projection. It might also be used to investigate the process in a therapeutic endeavor. Or it might be used to test parts of psychoanalytic propositions concerning personality and character.

For the isolated investigation of a basic psychoanalytic concept, I picked the concept of projection. Though repression was the basic defense mechanism of psychoanalytic theory until Anna Freud enlarged the list in her classic 1938 volume *The Ego and Its Mechanisms of Defense,* Freud had actually used the concept of projection as early as 1894 and 1896, and had used it extensively in his analysis of the Schreber Case, as the basic process of paranoia.

The concept of projection was generally formulated in American psychology as a defense mechanism in the service of the ego, designed in order to avoid awareness of unacceptable wishes, thoughts, and impulses, and accomplishing its task by ascribing such undesirable *subjective* phenomena to the *objective* world.

I attempted to demonstrate the process of projection by using the Thematic Apperception Test (TAT) (Bellak, 1950). In the experiment, some Harvard undergraduates were shown five pictures from the TAT under standard circumstances—and asked to tell a story about what was going on in the picture, what led up to it, and what the outcome would be. After the fifth picture, their performance was severely criticized. Then, after each subsequent picture and story (five in all), various criticisms were repeated.

The hypothesis underlying the experiment was that the criticism of their stories would enrage the subjects, and that they would not feel free to react with outward anger, but would instead "project" it and ascribe to the TAT pictures angry events that would be reflected in their responses. A simple word count confirmed that hypothesis.

I later had occasion to enlarge upon this technique, working with a group of seminary students in a training program for pastoral psychology at St. Elizabeth's Hospital in Washington, DC. Volunteers were hypnotized and given the posthypnotic suggestion to be angry, and then shown the second half of the pictures. Later, I repeated the experiment, telling the subjects to be depressed, with a similarly effective result. Finally, I suggested to one subject quite naively that he be happy in his posthypnotic stage, and indeed, in one of the subject's stories about TAT card #2, even the horse was smiling.

I gradually became aware of the fact that I had overreached myself. If projection was to be a defense mechanism, it made sense for subjects to "project" anger and depression, but why—unless it was inappropriate—did they project joy?

Following the suggestion of Ernst Kris, I rechecked Freud. Sure enough, in a frustrating footnote, Freud had anticipated that problem decades before my attempts: He viewed projection in a much broader sense, as a general perceptual process whereby all contemporary meaningful perception is predicated on and organized by the memory traces of all previous perceptions. By speaking of projection as part of the *continuum* of perception, Freud had made one tremendous step from a psychopathological concept to one pertaining to a general theory of personality. I therefore formulated the broader concept of *apperceptive distortion* in 1951, which I thought would be a more useful frame of reference for some of the so-called projective methods, although I can't say that the psychoanalytic literature had acted on that broadening of the concept of projection—or on any other. Decades later, academic psychology found it possible to acknowledge the role of affect in perception under the roof of *cognitive psychology*—a sort of backdoor admission of a basic psychoanalytic tenet to the previously barren brass instrument notation of perception.

With regard to the value of Freud's constructs concerning the causation of certain symptoms, of a neurotic or psychotic disturbance, of certain character structure and traits, some simple demonstration can be (in a strictly empirical sense) very impressive.

Sometimes, in seminars, I will ask a student to present only a patient's history, and will then encourage the rest of the class to predict what the symptoms and character structure ought to be. At other times, I will ask a student to relate only chief complaints and other symptoms of a patient, and have the rest postdict what crucial factors should have been present in the patient's childhood. In still another scenario, having heard the symptomatology, we try to infer what other problems a patient ought to have. This uncontrolled demonstration seems to work very well. But like so many psychoanalytic propositions, it has not yet been investigated with stringent, experimental precautions.

As we will discuss, the above clinical demonstration could easily be misleading with regard to the complexity of the task ahead; a multiplicity of assumptions and hypotheses underlie each inference we make. For instance, if the history reveals an unloving mother, it is not unreasonable to assume that the patient will have a tendency to depression. He will have this tendency because according to one of the psychoanalytic hypotheses, in order to have some healthy self-love and a good sense of self-esteem, one needs a loving figure (usually mother) to make one feel loved.

Mother's loving attitude is then "introjected," or internalized, so that one maintains an approving attitude toward oneself, even under adverse circumstances. If one is not that lucky, any reversal such as a job loss, an insult, or a rejection in love may cause a severe decrease in self-esteem and lead to a depression.

The process of internalization of images, attitudes, and so on has to be made explicit—possibly in terms of *Gestalten,* but not only visual ones. Harlow's experiments with his cloth monkeys, and Spitz's work on anaclitic depression and hospitalism, and more recent work by immunologists supporting the work of Harlow and Spitz suggest the importance of tactile sensations for the development of happiness, the avoidance of depression.

There are many more questions to be answered, hypotheses to be neatly stated and tested. For instance, we say, "A nonloving or rejecting or hostile mother is likely to lead to an unhappy, depressed child or adult." But just how unloving must a mother be to produce a depressed child, a depressed person? What is the critical cutoff point? Is there a formula to show *how little* love is necessary to produce a happy person?

Furthermore, how are we going to quantify? As I will suggest in Chapter One, we can use an ordinal scale, but it has yet to be constructed and tested.

Does rejection by a mother always lead to a depressed offspring? A great deal of mastery and competence on the part of the child could lead to a stable reaction formation, one that would not show depressive tendencies, even on projective tests. How can we predict that?

What else might a rejecting mother lead to? Instead of being primarily depressed, could the offspring of this mother be primarily unpleasant, angry, or vicious? What will it take to produce depression, what will it take to produce viciousness? Can there be a combination of these traits?

Surely there are many questions yet to be answered, but they are not unanswerable.

The simple assertion that a rejecting mother will lead to a depressed offspring involves psychoanalysis as a *learning theory:* The child learns not to expect love, not to love itself. It also involves psychoanalysis as a *perceptual theory:* How is the nonloving mother perceived and internalized? What kind of image is it—visual, tactile, auditory?

The same assertion also involves psychoanalysis as a *developmental theory:* We make the assumption that early learning (i.e., early in childhood), perhaps especially in the "oral" period, is intensively learned and of profound impact in the development of later personality. This assumption also involves the concept of "phase specificity," namely that oral experiences acquired in the oral period of development, and anal experiences learned in the "anal" period, are especially powerful formatively.

The concept of libidinal stages of development involves psychoanalysis as a developmental theory as well as psychoanalysis as an "economic" theory. In other words, there may be more or less "libidinal energy" invested in areas (erogenous zones) and aims (oral ingestion, genital union).

And with the *libido theory,* we have to deal with psychoanalysis as a *motivational theory.*

This enumeration just hints at the complexities to be stated neatly, laid out in a way that can be submitted to experimental verification or rejection. Indeed, such a process will be very valuable, if one then proceeds to psychoanalysis as a form of therapy and can improve the therapeutic work because of a better understanding of the nature of the hypotheses underlying the theory. This task involves a great deal of hard work, but it can be done—in spite of the complexities and obstacles involved in researching psychoanalysis.

Acknowledgments

Collaborating on a book is a marriage of sorts and can be almost as stressful. Therefore, I appreciate how painless and actually enjoyable it was to have James Walkup, Ph.D., as collaborator. His unusual erudition was a great asset. This does not mean we agreed throughout, however. The final responsibility is of course mine.

In a similar vein, Anne Herbst was that rare editor who did not get on the author's nerves. In addition, she was extremely helpful, especially when I hit snags, and brought intelligence and charm to the task.

Author's Note

All general gender references—"he," "him," "himself," and so on—have been masculinized for ease of expression, and reflect no bias on the part of the author.

CHAPTER ONE

Methodology

Introduction

Practically speaking, one of the most important facts about methodology is the attitudes people hold toward it. For far too long, methodology has been a no-man's-land, with opposing sides facing off against one another. Practicing analysts (mostly physicians until a recent lawsuit opened the doors to psychologists) have not usually been trained in research. Scientifically trained researchers, however, often lack firsthand experience as analysts; frequently they can do no better than guess—or find in books—meaningful units of the psychoanalytic work they are studying. But when research efforts are criticized by practicing analysts, researchers dismiss the criticisms as antiscientific prejudice.

Early in my career, I saw that the special circumstances of my background and training had prepared me to foster communication between the two sides. I am convinced that the distinction between loyalty to science and loyalty to clinical work is a false one. Of course, it is easy to make such noble statements; what counts is giving the conviction solidity through substantial, concrete work. While this has been no easy matter, it has allowed me to develop some rules of thumb for operating simultaneously in both camps.

Later, in Chapters Six and Seven, I will detail some successful applications of research methods to the problems of measuring ego functioning and studying clinical work. Let me anticipate these discussions by spelling out some of the issues involved.

A crucial problem with all psychoanalysis has been that of quantification. Psychoanalysts have traditionally shied away from quantitative statements because they felt that quantification was impossible. Although they might accept quantification of the lab values of drugs they prescribed, they considered it pseudoscientific when applied to psychoanalysis and therefore thoroughly misleading.

I believe psychoanalysts have felt this way because, like most people, they are accustomed to quantification only in scales such as the metric scale, characterized by equality of distance of the stops. My teacher, S. S. Stevens, taught me long ago that one can speak meaningfully of nominal, ordinal, and cardinal scales.

Ordinal scales can be useful in psychological measurement and can be usefully applied to psychoanalytic propositions. For instance, when we say that one person is more "anal," "oral," or "regressed" than another person, and less so than some third person, analysts might turn these judgments into simple quantitative comparative judgments, attributing one definition to each of the numbers. The number 7 might be defined as "quite anal" (excessively careful with money, extremely withholding, etc.) or "quite oral" (constantly hungry, constantly using multiple oral gratifications such as cigarettes, gum, candy). Other numbers could be similarly defined by gradations of the concept.

If we choose to operationalize, we might give these three people pictures of the Rorschach, utilizing lists of previously determined "anal," "oral," or "regressed" words, and count the number used by each person.

I have found the resistance that measurement has encountered surprising. An analyst will readily admit that a patient is currently showing almost no positive transference, that he was showing quite a bit of positive transference in the spring, and showed only a moderate amount over the summer. Yet that same analyst will be surprised when I say to him that these words can easily be turned into meaningful numbers, so that such comparisons take on increased precision.

What this analyst does not realize is that the branch of psychology often considered to be the most well established, and the closest to a natural science, is precisely the branch that regularly relies on judgments such as these. I have in mind sensation and perception, the branch in which Stevens made his greatest impact. Anyone who has been a subject in perception experiments knows that one is often asked comparative questions: Which light is brighter? Which figure seems farthest away? Which of these is heavier? and so on.

Some Basic Principles

I have always insisted that methodology is linked to conceptualization and, consequently, to broadly philosophical issues. Of course some of these issues are not unique to the psychoanalytic branch of science (e.g., causality). In the preceding example, in which someone makes a comparative judgment (of a percept or of a patient's transference), an essentially philosophical assumption is made that the two things being compared can be held in mind at the same time.

Every scientific concept is to some extent embedded in the framework of its philosophical assumptions. Typically these are implicit, not explicit. And, as my contact with logical positivism convinced me (see Chapter Seven), they are often related to the cultural milieu. This link to philosophical assumptions is as true of psychoanalysis as of other sciences. Problems in communication between psychoanalysis and philosophy will be discussed in Chapter Seven. For now, I shall illustrate this interrelation with three methodologically relevant basic principles: determinism, overdeterminism, and metapsychological principles.

Determinism

Although others had spoken of the mind deterministically, Freud was probably the first to do so in a truly thorough way: It was axiomatic that each behavioral act is determined by a specific cause or causes (and is itself a cause of other effects). His theory and practice of free association, for example, is based on the assumption of a causal connection that runs through unconscious motivations. And Freud's genetic viewpoint is a function of the consistent application of the law of causality to the shaping of the personality. (As I will discuss, my logical positivism has influenced me to see causality less as a "law" than as a resolution by the scientist to search for causes, and to believe that the search will not be in vain.)

The theory and practice of psychoanalysis is in fact predicated on determinism, though in my view this does not necessarily mean only rigid one-to-one relationships. Restatement in terms of probability theory is possible. Logically, once determinism has been accepted, the next step is to be concerned with the nature of the determining factors. They may be divided into two principal classes: sociopsychological-environmental determinants, and genetic-constitutional-prenatal-somatic-maturational ones. There are also countless complex interactions between these factors.

Determinism is a necessary assumption of therapy, predicated on the proposition that the contemporary "neurotic personality" is a result of early events and can be restructured.

Overdeterminism

Overdeterminism is but a special case of determinism—that a given event like a dream or a spoken sentence is the final common path of many genetically and contemporaneously derived forces. Strange as this concept may sound, it is of course also intrinsic to the physical world: The course of an object through space is determined by its weight, size, space, air currents, the impetus given, gravity, and so on, and the history of whether it was magnetized or exposed to a radioactive field. In one sense all forces—whether in psychiatry or physics—are contemporary ones; but for convenience of description and the best understanding of the interrelation of forces, a historical viewpoint can be adopted. Obviously the entire concept of "working through" is particularly predicated on the principle of overdeterminism.

Metapsychological Principles

The metapsychological principles themselves are predicated on the principle of determinism. Each psychological event, in order to be understood, must be examined from a dynamic, structural, and economic point of view. Since I am only concerned with illustrating how methods can be connected to basic principles, I will use the economic point of view as an illustration.

The economic assumptions are part of libido theory (see Chapter Five). Libido constitutes the energy of the system under study, and its cathexis in various libidinal aims and the countercathexis (in the defensive system) are basic forms of explanation. (*Cathexis* is a technical term that is equivalent to charge, investment, and attachment.) Implicitly, Freud considers each person as a closed energy system, to which the law of conservation of energy seems to apply; that is, if libido is withdrawn from one area, the psychoanalyst asks himself where it has been diverted or reinvested. This concept is fundamental to the theoretical understanding of narcissism and object-cathexis, and of symptom formation (though not any longer accepted by all psychoanalysts).

Consider, for example, the mechanistic application of the economic viewpoint in Freud's theories concerning wit, humor, and the comic. A certain conservation of energy previously used for repression is made available by the use of the trigger mechanisms of wit. The amount of energy is then "laughed off" and expended in somatic activity of the diaphragm and the facial muscles. Similarly, Freud conceives of humor as due to a conservation of energy for affective tone; he considers the pleasure of the comic as the conservation of energy incidental to the fact that the spectator feels he could perform the "comic" task with much less exertion than the comic does.

The problem of measurement may be simpler than it seems, if ordinal scaling techniques are used—certainly since their successful use in sensory psychology argues for their promise in such a project. In Chapter Four, I will offer my tentative schema for quantification of libido theory.

An Imaginary Operationalization

Earlier in this chapter, I stressed the practical importance of attitudes toward methodology, and in the last section of this chapter I will comment on this subject again. In the next two sections, I will illustrate my approach with two examples of large and, I believe, useful research projects for which I have been responsible. But before I turn to these, I want to try to bring home a point that is often left out of textbooks that discuss methodology. Specifically, I believe an insufficiently appreciated contribution to useful methodology is the capacity to regress slightly, in the sense of Ernst Kris's "adaptive regression in the service of the ego," allowing the imagination to enter into the serious business of science.

Let me illustrate this sort of intermingling by continuing my discussion of economic factors. Consider two well-known propositions of the development of libidinal cathexis. The first object is usually understood to be the infant's own body, which is as yet undifferentiated from the world. This first state is designated narcissistic. The second type of object choice is described as an anaclitic object choice (*anaclitic* means "leaning against"). The child relates first to that figure who supplies him with gratification of his needs, and only the final achievement of cathexis of a person outside the family is considered true object-cathexis.

The economic implications here involve the idea that the amount of libido that was originally invested in the self is decreased by the amount invested, say, in the mother figure. Imagine baby John started out with a total narcissistic investment of libido of 100,000 Freudian units. He may be investing 20,000 units in the mother. Thereupon baby John would be left only with 80,000 Freudian units with which to keep house. John may be expected to invest some of this in his father, his brothers and sisters, his teachers, and others. (Incidentally, according to another proposition never quite explicitly stated, John can never go completely bankrupt.) Some units always stay invested in John's body and in various libidinal zones. Some units are intricately bound up in his defenses and countercatheses and his intrapsychic system as a whole.

John's progress in libidinal object choices could very well be traced quantitatively. Consider the well-known resolution of the oedipal constellation, which is frequently discussed. John has invested 20,000 units in his mother as the object of his aim for genital (and other) gratification. He also has considerable investment in his penis. Say the penis has received 300,000 units of investment. John fears he will lose it, plus his investment in his father, if he does not forgo (or withdraw) the investment in his mother. To put it mildly, this would be bad business.

John can resolve the dilemma by withdrawing 15,000 from his mother and changing the nature of his financial ambitions from one of primary control over the mother to one of sympathetic, token participation. He reinvests some of the units in the superego (those internal police forces that should protect him from getting so far out on a limb again) and some in his father (making friends with an enemy who, once discovered to be valiant, has become admired). He keeps the bulk of his libido as ready working capital for a series of transactions.

Ultimately, John is expected to withdraw a considerable sum of units—say 15,000 of the 20,000 units originally invested in the mother, and some 5,000 of those invested in the sister, and an equal amount from those invested in brother and father—and now briefly but richly endow a series of girlfriends and finally settle 30,000 units on his wife, at least during the courtship. This amount is to be further increased by, say, 10,000 units from his own narcissistic reserves.

When the stork arrives and John has his first child, it will be time for further reinvestment from the family, from his narcissistic pool, and possibly from the original heated investment in his wife. These funds will be put in the newly opened account, his baby. As he lives on he can be expected to decrease his narcissistic supply to the safe minimum necessary for intact operation, self-protection, and self-esteem—much as any good business adventure will not let the reserves be depleted below a certain minimum. At the same time, for maximal health, all expendable units should be freely circulating, expended on his family, friends, community, and work.

This is of course a fantasized version of a serious scientific story, yet it has a point. It allows many presuppositions to become explicit. Although I have not myself derived specific experiments from this account, it can be a useful cognitive detour that facilitates experimental formulations. (For example, it might be possible to have subjects set quantitative figures on choices between imaginary states of affairs—such as a visit from Mom versus avoiding a row with Dad.) And, because it dramatizes the components of the model, the researcher is in a better position to find the most appealing option.

In the next two sections, I use illustrative material from later chapters to describe two examples of major research projects that have combined derivation of hypotheses from psychoanalytic principles, clinically meaningful units of measurement, and flexible research methodologies.

Example One: Ego Assessment

In Chapter Six, I describe in detail the development of a now widely used technique for ego function assessment. In this chapter, I will anticipate this discussion by illustrating some of my practices regarding the extraction of clinically meaningful units and the application of research methodology.

I believe the psychoanalyst-clinician must make a decisive break from the commonsense notion of the ego as "the I" or the unitary self as a source of agency and perspective. Instead, psychoanalytic theory and practice must assume that, despite the unitary appearance of the ego, it can be understood as being composed of and defined by various functions. In treatment, this allows the analyst (1) to address technically various impairments in functioning by interpreting sources of conflict that cause problems and (2) where necessary, to support enfeebled or insufficiently developed functions.

The researcher should follow the lead of the clinician here. If the ego is defined by its functions, one can investigate experimentally how well it performs the functions (i.e., design tests for reality testing, frustration and anxiety tolerance, rigidity, motor functions, etc.). Still, although the ego is not unitary, the assessment of ego strength needs to be global, much as intelligence is understood to be on the Wechsler system. Global evaluation is needed because sometimes one ego function can substitute for another.

When I set out to design a method of ego function assessment, I traced the theoretical development of the term. Twelve ego functions were selected (for a fuller description, see Chapter Six). The most natural way to evaluate the ego functions was to use the traditional clinical interview (though it has proven possible to apply this method to other types of data, such as psychotherapy sessions). The interview was used, but it was necessary to introduce checks on reliability and to provide quantitative methods of comparison. A manual was therefore written, with a scale provided for each ego function. On one form, the numbers ran from 1 (poor or minimal functioning) to 13 (optimal), with 11 as the "average" functioning (understood as something short of optimal functioning, but without significant psychopathology). (Another form used a scale of 1–7.)

Labeling end points is not really exact enough, however, so detailed descriptions were written for the odd-numbered points on the scale. Also, each function was itself understood to have components and each component was rated individually. (For example, one ego function is called "regulation and control of drives, affects, and impulses." The interviewer rates each component, one concerning the directness of the expression of an impulse, the other having to do with the effectiveness of the delay and control exercised by the patient.)

The great advantage of using this approach is that profiles of an individual can be constructed so that he can be compared to others and to his own functioning at different times. The scientist and clinician are better able to make predictions, present histories, and the like. (And, not incidentally, those wishing to justify funding for various types of treatment are able to have more objective modes of description available to them.)

Naturally, if such a system captures the construct of ego functioning, one would usually expect that persons who have different levels of ego functioning would, on the average, produce different scores. And indeed, in a NIMH-sponsored study I conducted with my colleagues, we found that the mean score for normals was 9.08; for neurotics, 7.42; and for schizophrenics, 5.86. Although this does not prove the validity of the system, we would not have had much confidence in our manual had the differences failed to emerge.

Also, the manual would produce misleading comparisons if raters used it in different ways. Fortunately, we found that interrater reliability between judges who used the specially designed manual to evaluate an individual ranged from 0.61 for the "stimulus barrier" ego function to 0.88 for the "autonomous functioning" ego function. Even the lower of these two scores is pretty good as these things go, and we later found that ordinary psychotherapy sessions could be rated with a reliability of 0.72.

Example Two: Psychotherapy

In Chapter Eight, I describe in detail how I organized an attempt to study empirically the actual conduct of an analysis. Today, it may be difficult for the reader to imagine the resistance this attempt encountered, for it was thought impossible or inappropriate by many practicing analysts.

In this case, I found it necessary to draw on and (where possible) improve many of the cognitive activities that take place in the analyst's mind. These activities are often quasi-scientific and, with a little help, can be brought out into the open and used to transform private intuitions into publicly demonstrable data.

Let me illustrate: Consider a mild obsessive-compulsive disorder. The clinical analyst's first step is often to formulate a very general hypothesis. Without knowing more than that this man suffers from an obsessive-compulsive disorder, using various basic principles, the analyst reasons that a conflict is at work between aggression and the superego. He might tentatively hypothesize that the ego alien neurotic features will probably coexist with some ego-syntonic ones of compulsive character traits. Furthermore, the analyst will reason, these traits are generally consistent with propositions pertaining to anal personality traits used as a defense against aggression (e.g., retentiveness, neatness, tightness, etc.).

Next, problems of methodology surface as problems of technique. Assuming that the above hypothesis is borne out by what the patient has to say (which, we assume, includes a history consistent with an anal personality), the analyst will decide on areas of interventions, methods of intervention (clarification, interpretation, etc.), and sequences of intervention. The first area might be a conflict between his wish to socialize and his anger over spending money. Or the analyst might offer an interpretation of his fear of being poor like his father, his wish to do better, and his guilt over this wish. In the future—and in the back of the analyst's mind—there might be the interpretation of his wish to do better for his mother than his father had done, or the conflict between his being successful and his wish to remain a dependent and adored child of his mother.

Obviously, methodological considerations have already entered the picture, although in this case methodology is understood as a treatment technique or a tool. If we proceed to the next level, which is to prove the veracity of the hypothesis concerning the origin of the patient's symptoms, a new (but not unrelated) sense of methodology arises. Independent observation must be used, with outside observers reviewing the clinical material. A format must be devised so that the judgments of the observers are comparable. This requires quantification.

In this process, nets of collateral inference are constructed. These include predictions concerning future material that will arise in response to interpretations, and also postdictions (reconstructions of the past) regarding as yet unknown material from the patient's history.

Along with some colleagues, I arranged for the tape recording and transcription of analyses. A group of analysts was assembled to evaluate and judge the clinical material. One group was responsible for making predictions, while others judged the session material itself. Transcripts were distributed weekly and predictions made regarding the upcoming time frame (next session, next week, next month). Forms were prepared and ratings made. Regular meetings were conducted and, overall, strong correlations were held for the ratings performed.

Others have since picked up where we left off, but I feel we were successful in demonstrating the viability of this sort of work. And, most importantly, we found that a scientific project could be organized around many of the already existing modes of clinical inference and that these could be improved without serious distortion.

Methodology and the Mundane

More attention should be paid to the mundane aspects of methodology. Psychological research is now several generations old and yet, with very few exceptions, little use has been made of the storehouse of data collected so far. This is partly because tastes change and new measures are developed, but more should be done to find ways this state of affairs can usefully be exploited.

Data collection should, whenever possible, aim to code the data in forms that make it available to other (sometimes competing) research teams. This would help eliminate the argument "My sample was different from your sample." At least until the field has developed standardized constructs that are likely to last, an effort should be made to code data in some relatively generic terms, which allow those with alternative assumptions to utilize them. Wherever possible, archives of tape recordings and videotaped material should be easily accessible to other researchers.

I hope that psychoanalytic institutes, which are currently in the midst of many changes, will now make a renewed effort to provide a prominent place for research training in the curriculum. Such a training program makes a statement to new candidates about the scientific commitments of the discipline. Even those clinicians who will never be involved in research can become intelligent and discerning consumers of the research of others—and will, I believe, leave them less likely to adhere dogmatically to ideas that have failed to gain support from the data. I think a concerted effort to produce first-rate psychoanalytic researchers is an absolutely fundamental requirement if psychoanalysis is to have a productive future.

I began this chapter with a comment on the practical importance of people's attitudes toward methodology. I shall close with a related comment. Some aspects of methodology are mundane. They lack the psychological drama of clinical work and the eager excitement of uncovering new discoveries in research. But they are necessary and, rightly understood, they can be enjoyable for their own sake.

It is important for the methodologist to cultivate, to the greatest possible extent, a pleasure in devising a neat solution to a technical problem. For some reason, many intellectuals have a distaste for the work of the craftsman or the technician.

What fascinates me is the sheer ingenuity needed to develop a clever method of doing a good, efficient job. Consider the ice cream cone, which manages to double as both a container and as part of the snack; or the "lazy Susan," a revolving circular platform that allows easy access to items at the back of a cabinet; or the newly developed lightweight jacket that can be folded tightly into its hood and zipped shut, allowing the wearer to carry it in a pocket.

Historically, this "Yankee ingenuity" has been associated with Americans. Although Benjamin Franklin was a statesman and something of a political thinker, he took pride in his inventions, such as bifocal glasses, the Franklin stove, and others. Thomas Jefferson's house, Monticello, is filled with brilliant technological innovations.

The psychoanalyst who is willing to get his hands a bit dirty by fiddling with scales, predictions, and the like can not only expect to contribute to science but, with a little Yankee ingenuity, may expect to have some fun, too.

CHAPTER TWO

Psychoanalytic Theory of Personality as Learning Theory

Introduction

Psychoanalysts try to obtain as careful and detailed a history of their patients as possible. In my own teaching, I insist on knowing not only a patient's history from birth but also any prenatal conditions of the mother and fetus. I also try to have a clear conceptualization of where the patient was born, how the apartment or house looked, what the prevailing atmosphere in the home was, whether there were siblings and what were their age relationships to the patient, who slept where and with whom, and the like. Other details of the patient's profile include his performance in school, his relation to his teachers and his peers, and so on, up to the present. Most other psychoanalysts also engage in this kind of inquiry for this reason: *We think implicitly of behavior as learned, and of psychoanalysis as a very specific kind of learning theory.*

When eliciting a patient's chief complaint, I insist on similarly exhaustive detail and specificity (i.e., not just the year or month the problem started but preferably the exact day and time). I also want to know about the life situation or circumstances at the time the complaint started or escalated, and every other detail. I engage in this process because I believe that the precipitating situation will share common denominators with earlier situations in the patient's life, and so he repeats a coping mechanism, even if maladaptive, that he has "learned" earlier.

It is possible that *in-utero* emotional and physical experiences other than genetic factors have already affected the fetus, by imprint or learning. From the very first few hours of caring for the infant, experience will translate itself into psychological structure. The infant "learns" to expect overstimulation or sensory deprivation, as Spitz has shown. We know tentatively from the work by Fries and Woolf that if a mother holds her infant too tightly or too awkwardly, the child is likely to be irritable, having "learned" to expect the world to be uncomfortable.

Furthermore, psychoanalysis as learning theory suggests that if a child has shared the parental bed and frequently witnessed sexual relations between the parents, he may have learned to fear the alarming noises and movements. Such children may learn to cope in different ways, depending on circumstances and possibly on their autonomous functions, such as intelligence and mastery competence, and on some biological factors, such as stimulation barriers. Some may "learn" to be withdrawn and to avoid overstimulation in their later life, or may even become recluses. Conversely others may always require overstimulation and affective-behavioral discharge through nervousness, overwork, and hypomanic behavior.

Some children may learn to deal with what psychoanalysts call the "primal scene" by running away from home, sleeping in the attic, or moving out of the house as soon as possible. And some may develop defenses such as denial, or may repress the disturbing experiences and not recall them in adult life. In any case, we may frequently find that the adult has repeated nightmares of being attacked.

Psychoanalysis as learning theory also suggests that certain functions that have been "learned," such as bowel and bladder control, may be unlearned again under certain traumatic circumstances. I recall a 7-year-old boy who was brought to me for a consultation because he had recently started to have violent nightmares and to wet his bed. It turned out that all this had started a few weeks earlier when he had to give up his little room and bed to an impecunious aunt. He then had to share a bed with his mother and father. Thinking the boy was asleep, they often engaged in sexual relations. He was in fact awake enough to be both frightened, as shown by the nightmares, and overstimulated, as evidenced by the bed wetting which, as a form of release, resulted in loss of sphincter control.

In the case of the bed wetting, we may speak of regressing from a later learned sphincter control or use of the bathroom, to an earlier way of behaving or coping with a full bladder. Psychoanalysts call such behavior *regressive*. Yet, in their own way, these symptoms are also forms of coping, and the dreams are a form of problem solving. The problems of this boy were easily resolved by my suggestion that the mother get a sleeping bag for the kitchen floor and let the boy sleep there. His symptoms quickly abated.

It is possible that this boy, when grown up, may approach sexual situations with an anxiety recalling the parental bed. When it is time for him to ejaculate during intercourse, he will probably experience a urination-like premature ejaculation, again a fearful regression to the childhood symptomatology.

We will later discuss the experimental exploration of regression of learned behavior. Meanwhile, it is important to stress that people may cope in different ways with a seemingly identical experience or situation. It remains one of the challenges of experimental study to see what hidden determinants such as age, temperament of the parents, or ethnic factors can be found for these different coping mechanisms. For instance, I once saw a middle-aged man who suffered a severe coronary infarction and was sent for a psychiatric evaluation and recommendation for rehabilitation. His history revealed a prolonged sharing of the parental bed. His dreams revealed fears of passivity, some of which could be considered fear of homosexual attack. In his manifest life, he presented himself as the prototypical "tough guy." As a bus driver, he prided himself on doing his route in a shorter time than anyone else. His coronary occurred while he was working as a truck driver, driving as well as loading and unloading—and in record time and weight.

I believe that this man must have experienced a great deal of passivity as a child, which he perceived as a fear of being molested, invaded, and "raped" like his mother. He coped in early adolescence by being extra tough, and maintained this behavior pattern in his occupation to cope with that initial fear of passivity. His learned behavior might verbally be stated: "It is not true that I am afraid of being helpless against intrusion. The truth is that I am a tough guy who can beat anyone in the house."

This is a simple example of character structure as a form of *learned coping behavior*. There are infinitely more complex character formations.

Oedipus Simplified

The embattled oedipus complex is a central concept of psychoanalysis. As such, it has been mythologized and overemphasized in importance, but it has also been inappropriately dismissed.

In its basest form, the oedipus complex proposes that the son has a desire to possess his mother and to get his father out of the way. Character formation is then a learned form of coping with the resulting constellation and symptomatology. I suggest that we see the oedipus situation simply as two parties competing for the same object. The son is usually weaker and faces (among other obstacles) an alliance between the parents. (This may not always be true, as in the case of the mother who demeans her husband and makes the son the man of her dreams.)

The young man may try to solve the triangular situation by saying, "This is a dangerous, no-win situation and I give up." His solution may be to become passive, and under certain circumstances of complete surrender, a homosexual—who will either be the passive object vis-à-vis another or, identifying with the father, will be a sadist toward other males.

Another son, attempting to deal with his anxiety, may be rebellious as a boy, a troublemaker in school, and openly rebellious against his father. He will accept beatings rather than submit quietly, and may be angry at authority figures for the rest of his life.

Under more fortunate circumstances, the oedipus complex may be resolved as the boy identifies with the father and cedes him the mother in the initial contest, but soon finds a female love object of his own.

In all the above cases, we are dealing with learned behavior as a means of dealing with conflicts and as a form of conflict-resolution, or a way of coping. We can speak of healthy coping, as opposed to lack of coping or neurotic, self-harming, pathological coping.

One of the best known and fairly frequent pathological outcomes of the oedipal constellation manifests itself in what psychoanalysts refer to as a "success neurosis." There are people, more often men than women, who seem to be intelligent and competent but always manage to fail in life's endeavors. Upon exploration, it often turns out that they are afraid of competing with the internalized father, and now unconsciously equate all success with symbolically succeeding in winning the mother. As adults, these people will often create a condition that ensures that they will not succeed vocationally. One man whom I treated had a lifelong recurring nightmare in which he tried to get through a narrow channel and failed to do so because of various dire impediments. The love canal was too dangerous a passage for him.

I believe that in each instance of character structure and symptomatology, it is possible to state the psychoanalytic propositions in the form of hypotheses that can lend themselves to simple operational statements and experimental exploration.

As discussed in Chapter One, the method of prediction,

postdiction, and collateral inferences is my favorite tool of investigation. I would also draw on large tape libraries of recorded psychoanalytic sessions in order to make inferences based on data from large numbers of patients with similar histories and/or pathology. Experimental analogues, like that of Mowrer's study of regression, Sears's study of projection in college students, or my study of projection, are examples of other possible forms of researching psychoanalytic concepts. Yet, though such experimental exploration is possible, it still has not been carried out to the necessary degree. Psychoanalysts are simply not aware of many of the implicit assumptions they make—and that these assumptions relate to long-established "laws" of academic psychology. Without ever saying so explicitly or systematically, psychoanalysts believe that the earlier in a person's life something happened, the more lasting structural effect it will have. Similarly, it is held that a person is likely to have a worse effect from repeated traumas than from one trauma. The first is an example of the *law of primacy,* the second of the *law of frequency.*

The validity of the law of primacy, which is implicit in psychoanalytic theory, could be investigated by finding x number of subjects who suffered separation in infancy and childhood. These subjects would have to be matched (more or less) for severity of circumstances involved in a separation and other factors. They would also have to be the same age at the time of the investigation, and would have to have suffered separation at different ages. With these and all other factors controlled, the hypothesis to be proven is that the subjects who suffered separation earlier will evidence more severe pathology than those who suffered separation at a later date. (Severity is defined by a set of acceptable criteria.)

A similar design could be used for the law of frequency, with other factors being matched. Those who have been abused or rejected more frequently should show more pathology than those who were traumatized less often.

To pick a different aspect of "learning" in psychoanalytic theory, consider the role of learning to cope. One learns different and presumably better mechanisms for coping as one grows up. Current developmental psychoanalytic research (e.g., by Lichtenberg and Beebe) carefully describes the processes observed.

One experimental study of a defense mechanism as a demonstration of learning was long ago performed by Mowrer and Ullman, who produced an experimental analogue of regression. First, rats were trained to learn to turn off any painful electric stimulus by pushing a lever with their noses. Then this effect was made inoperable; they learned that if they stood on their hind legs the electric stimulation would be turned off. After a while Mowrer changed the rules again, and the rats learned that standing on their hind legs did not help to shut off the painful current. He then observed that the rats returned to pushing the lever with their noses.

Perceptual Learning

According to classical theory, and particularly to object relation theory, a child learns certain kinds of object relations in part by conditioning. The child expects what he has learned before from a new situation and internalizes an introject, such as percepts of a loving mother or a punishing mother. These internalized object representations then determine future object choice, such as marrying or rejecting a woman who is similar to the mother. Indeed, future perception of objects are influenced by previously "learned" ones.

The same holds true for object representations. Projective techniques lend themselves ideally to demonstration of the effect of past percepts on contemporary perception.

In the Thematic Apperception Test (TAT), picture #1 shows a young boy sitting behind a violin. When subjects are asked to relate a story about that picture, they tell an infinite variety of stories. A relatively popular one is of a boy who was told to practice by his mother but would rather play ball with the other children outside. The attitude ascribed to the parent usually reflects accurately how the subject perceived his parent. How he deals with this conflict between parental authority and his own desires reflects itself in the story. Some smash the violin and play football, eventually making All American; others, by not obeying the parent, become bums and regret their disobedience all their lives; still others practice the violin and, as a reward for their obedience, become soloists at Carnegie Hall.

A more complex story relates how the violin is broken and no sound comes from it, reflecting the damage to the subject's own self-image. Yet another subject does not perceive a violin at all, but rather a sword in its case. This person is so permeated with aggression, feeling it and fearing it, that the violin is not seen at all. The instrument of music in this case becomes an instrument of aggression.

In the Children's Apperception Test (CAT), when the subjects are shown a picture of a lion and a mouse, they tell stories of the mouse who helps the lion so that they become good friends. Alternatively, the lion chases the mouse, who disappears into its hole; in pursuit, the lion bumps his head and dies. These stories obviously reflect quite different object representations and self-representations.

Even without pictures a great deal may be learned. For years I have simply asked people to look at a blank wall and imagine a picture. Not only will the choice of picture be very informative but the subject's story about the imaginary picture will be highly indicative. To pick a simple case, one man imagined a beautiful island scene with palm trees, gentle waves, and a boat. Unfortunately, as in a painting by Utrillo, there were no human beings in the setting, suggesting the withdrawn, narcissistic nature of the artist.

In dreams, too, many things can be very obviously reflected and understood as self and object representations. For instance, one Vietnam veteran had been repeatedly disturbed by a dream in his childhood of a giant gorilla chasing him. Now it was more often a case of Viet Cong *guerrillas* attacking in his nocturnal dream. It was not difficult for him to become aware of the fact that his mother was the threatening gorilla of his childhood, and the guerrillas were the more recently perceived threat of the Viet Cong superimposed on the earlier feared mother, who had often beaten him painfully.

I investigated this matter of *apperceptive distortion*, a term I prefer to *projection* in such a case, in a series of experiments. (See my discussion of the TAT in the Introduction.)

Of the three principal structures in psychoanalytic theory of personality—the *id, ego,* and *superego*—the ego and superego are, in different ways and for different purposes, the repository of learning. These structures will be discussed in detail in Chapter Four.

Of the 12 ego functions that I have found to be both necessary and sufficient to describe personality, two are outstandingly based on previous learning: reality testing and judgment. The child learns, in this case largely through conditioning and trial and error, that there is a feedback (or proprioception) from his own body but not from other objects. In psychoanalytic psychopathology, the fact of insufficient learning about the body image leads to disorders such as poor self-boundaries and symbiosis which, as Jacobson and Federn pointed out, are important in depression and schizophrenia. Sechehaye (1955) described the case of a completely depersonalized girl, whom she painstakingly taught for years to acquire self-boundaries by stroking different parts of her body.

Figure drawing, for diagnostic purposes, often dramatically illustrates disturbances of the body image (e.g., pathology of body image). An adolescent boy may be revealed to see himself as a little girl, and somebody else may draw stiff arms without hands, perhaps indicating either difficulties with social contact or conflict about masturbation.

All information about the world is *learned,* from the simple fact that some objects are too hot to be touched, to the complex rules of the social game. Thus reality testing and judgment are learned functions. In different cultures, different rules are learned concerning what is real and what is not. When a Russian colleague attempted to construct a reality testing scale, he devised items such as what to do when one notices oneself followed by a black limousine or finds oneself suddenly without any kind of document. These items required completely different reality testing and judgment than those I would have derived.

Psychoanalysts, to be sure, have numerous different propositions concerning learning and the superego. They think of bowel sphincter training as related to the acquisition of mores. *Thou shalt not be dirty* becomes part of the decalogue. Severe cleanliness training may then "teach" a child obsessive cleanliness, as well as overly severe morality. The initial "Don't get dirty!" can be expanded to include all impulse control. Of course, in its role as the conscience, the superego is mainly the conscious part of the personality and is the repository of social learning in general, including such distinctions as what is or is not fair play.

A few very specific learning propositions are involved in the conceptualization of drives, subsumed in psychoanalytic theory under the construct of the id.

The libido theory, intricately related to learning theory in its form and developmental theory, involves the concept of *phase specificity*. This concept states that oral experiences, when acquired in the oral period, will be more effectively learned, and therefore will have more of a structuring effect on the personality than if they were learned in the anal or phallic period of development. A practical aspect of this hypothesis in psychopathology is the assumption that the starvation of an infant during the oral phase will lead to more severe pathology than if it had occurred in some other phase of development where different issues are more prominent. In the oral phase, the starvation experience might result in the need to overeat and in fantasies as well as impulses to gorge oneself. These impulses in turn might lead to severe problems of overall impulse control.

Both longitudinal studies and process studies in enough recorded cases could easily test these analytic propositions and, more specifically, the psychopathological ones.

CHAPTER THREE

Psychoanalysis as a Perceptual Theory

Introduction

In the history of philosophy, Hume wrote *Nihil est in intellectu quid none antea fuerit in sensibus* ("Nothing is in the mind that has not previously been in the senses"), and Berkeley wrote *Esse est percipi* ("To be is to perceive"). There can be little doubt that perception structures the personality. Within psychoanalysis, developmentalists like to discuss good development in terms of the differentiation of the self and its relation to the object world, a perceptual process.

In my view, none of the schools of psychoanalysis speaks concretely and clearly enough of perception to eliminate the arcane and unnecessarily abstract terminology. As I conceptualize it, each visual perception is retained in a kaleidoscopic tube. Each subsequent transparency has to be seen through the first one, and each subsequent perception, whether the tenth perception or the hundred-thousandth, is seen through a screen of all the previous ones. If, for instance, mother is seen in 10 different images, the resultant *gestalt* or configuration has features of all of them, but constitutes a unique *gestalt* or configuration itself. The complexity of personality can be understood in terms of this tremendous number of "transparencies."

In turn, the process of analyzing these transparencies on the couch is necessarily a lengthy one; at best only a few regnant *gestalten* can be analyzed or isolated from the mass. By learning from the transference and by other interpretations, the unconscious *gestalt* of mother acquired in childhood may be altered by interpolating adult, contemporary views of her. These can be arrived at with the help of both the adult intelligence of the patient and the analyst's interpretation.

In the next sections, I extend my treatment by reintroducing the concept of apperception and show how it can be understood within the framework of psychoanalysis. At the end of the chapter, I will elaborate on some of the consequences of my approach for viewing familiar clinical phenomena.

Perception and Apperception

I speak of apperception as an organism's (dynamically) meaningful interpretation of a perception. This definition evolved in German philosophy, and its direct source is the definition by C. P. Herbart in his *Psychologie als Wissenschaft* (Part III, Section I, Chapter 5, p. 15) as quoted in Dagobert D. Runes, editor of the *Dictionary of Philosophy*: "Apperception (Latin, *ad* plus *percipere* to perceive) in psychology: The process by which new experience is assimilated to and transformed by the residuum of past experience of any individual to form a new whole. The residuum of past experience is called apperceptive mass."

This definition and the use of the term *apperception* permit us to suggest, as a working hypothesis, that there can be a hypothetical process of noninterpreted perception, and that every subjective interpretation constitutes a dynamically meaningful apperceptive distortion. Conversely, we can also establish, operationally, a condition of nearly pure cognitive "objective" perception in which a majority of subjects agree on the exact definition of a stimulus. For instance, the majority of subjects agree that picture #1 of the TAT shows a boy sitting behind a violin. We can thus establish this perception as a norm, and say that anyone who, for instance, describes this picture as a boy at a lake (as one schizophrenic patient did) distorts the stimulus situation apperceptively. If we let any of our subjects go on to further description of the stimulus, however, we find that each one of them interprets the stimulus differently—as a happy boy, a sad boy, an ambitious boy, a boy urged on by his parents, and so on. We must therefore state that purely cognitive perception remains a construct and that every person distorts apperceptively, the distortions differing only in degree.

In the clinical use of the TAT it becomes quite clear that we deal with apperceptive distortions of varying degrees (Bellak, forthcoming). The subject is frequently unaware of any subjective significance in the story he tells. It has been found in clinical practice that simply asking the subject to read over his typewritten story may often give him sufficient distance from the situation to perceive that the gross aspects of it refer to himself. Only after considerable psychotherapy, however, is he able to see his more latent drives; and he may never be able to "see" the least acceptable of his subjective distortions, although they are detected by any number of independent observers. It may be permissible, then, to introduce a number of terms of apperceptive distortion of varying degree for purposes of identification and communication. (Bear in mind that these various forms of apperceptive distortion do not necessarily exist in pure form and often patently coexist with each other.)

Forms of Apperceptive Distortion

Inverted Projection

It is suggested that the term *projection* be reserved for the greatest degree of apperceptive distortion, such as paranoid delusions. Its opposite pole would be, hypothetically, a completely objective perception. Projection was originally described in clinical psychoanalysis as pertaining to certain neurotic defenses generally, to psychoses in particular, and to some "normal" maturational processes. We may say that in the case of true projection we are dealing not only with an ascription of feelings and sentiments that remain unconscious but that are unacceptable to the ego and are therefore ascribed to objects of the outside world. We may also add that they cannot be made conscious except by special prolonged therapeutic techniques.

This concept encompasses the phenomenon observed in a paranoid, which can be essentially stated as the change from the unconscious "I love him" to the conscious "He hates me." True projection in this case is actually a very complex process, probably involving the following four steps: (1) "I love him" (a homosexual object)—an unacceptable id drive; (2) "I hate him"—reaction formation; (3) the aggression is also unacceptable and is repressed; and (4) finally, the percept is changed to "He hates me." On the last step, this feeling of "He hates me" usually reaches consciousness.

I suggest calling this process *inverted* projection, as contrasted with simple projection, which is discussed below. The first step in the process usually involves the operation of another defense mechanism, reaction formation. It is sufficient to say here that, in the case of the paranoid, "I hate him" is approved, whereas "I love him" (homosexually) is socially disapproved; he learned it early as a dangerous impulse in relation to his father. In this case, "I hate him" extinguishes and replaces the loving sentiment. Thus in inverted projection we first deal with the process of reaction formation, and then with an apperceptive distortion that results in the ascription of the subjective sentiment to the outside world as a simple projection.

Simple Projection

This mechanism is not necessarily of clinical significance, but occurs frequently. The following joke describes it well:

Joe Smith wants to borrow Jim Jones's lawnmower. As he walks across his own lawn he thinks of how he will ask Jones for the lawnmower. But then he thinks: "Jones will say that the last time I borrowed something from him I gave it back dirty." Smith answers him in fantasy by replying that it was in the same condition in which he had received it. Then Jones replies in fantasy by saying that Smith will probably damage Jones's fence as he lifts the mower over. Whereupon Smith replies . . . and so the fantasy argument continues. When Joe finally arrives at Jim's house, Jim stands on the porch and says cheerily, "Hello, Joe, what can I do for you?" and Joe responds angrily, "You can keep your damn lawnmower!"

Broken down simply, this story means the following: Joe wants something but recalls a previous rebuff. He has learned (from parents, siblings, etc.) that the request may not be granted. This makes him angry. He then perceives Jim as angry with him, and his response to the imagined aggression is: "I hate Jim because Jim hates me."

In greater detail, this process can be seen as follows: Joe wants something from Jim. This brings up the image of asking something from another contemporary—his brother, for example, who is seen as jealous and would angrily refuse in such a situation. Thus the process might simply be: The image of Jim is apperceptively distorted by the percept memory of the brother, a case of inappropriate transfer of learning. I will attempt later to explain why Joe does not relearn if reality proves his original conception wrong. The empirical fact is established that such neurotic behavior does not usually change except under psychotherapy.

Joe differs from the paranoid in several ways—by the lesser rigidity with which he adheres to his projections; by less frequency and less exclusiveness; and by the smaller degree of his lack of awareness, or inability to become aware of how patently subjective and absurd the distortion is.

Consider this recurring scenario: A person arrives late for work on Monday morning and believes, incorrectly, that his supervisor looks angrily at him later in the day. This is spoken of as "a guilty conscience"; that is, he behaves as though the supervisor knew that he had come late, when, in reality, the supervisor may not know it at all. The person sees in the supervisor the anger that he has come to expect from such a situation. Again, this behavior can be understood as a simple (associative) distortion through transfer of learning, or, in more complex situations, the influence of previous images on present ones. (See Bellak, 1944, on evidence regarding projection.)

Sensitization

Let us modify the above case. If we now have a situation in which the supervisor feels a very slight degree of anger at the latecomer, we may observe a new phenomenon. Some people may not notice the anger at all and thus not react to it, whereas others may both notice and react to it. In the latter case, we shall find that these people are the ones who tend to perceive anger even at times when it does not objectively exist. This well-known clinical fact has been spoken of as the "sensitivity" of neurotics. Instead of the creation of an objectively nonexistent percept, we now deal with a more sensitive perception of existing stimuli. (A very similar process has been described by Eduardo Weiss as *objectivation*.) The hypothesis of sensitization merely means that an object that fits a preformed pattern is more easily perceived than one that does not fit the preformed pattern. This fact is widely accepted, as in the perceptual problems of reading, wherein previously learned words are much more easily perceived by their pattern than by their spelling.

Sensitization, I believe, is also the process that took place in the experiment by Levine, Chein, and Murphy (1943). When these experimenters first starved a number of subjects and then fleetingly showed them pictures that depicted (among other things) objects of food, they found two processes: When starved, (1) the subjects saw food in the fleeting pictures even if there was none and (2) the subjects correctly perceived actual pictures of food more frequently. Apparently in such a state of deprivation there is an increased cognitive efficiency of the ego in recognizing objects that might obviate its deprivation, and also a simple compensatory fantasy of wish fulfillment, which the authors call *autistic perception*. Thus the organism is equipped for both reality adjustment and substitutive gratification where real gratification does not exist. This reaction represents an increase in the efficiency of the ego's function in response to an emergency—a more accurate perception of food when the subject is in the state of starvation. I believe that this process can also be subsumed under our concept of sensitization, since food images are recalled by the starvation and real food stimuli are more easily perceived.

Autistic Perception

Whether the perception of desired food objects in the state of starvation among stimuli that do not objectively represent food objects constitutes a form of simple projection, or is a process that should be described as distinct from it depends on rather fine points. We may see that the increased need for food leads to a recall of food objects, and that these percept memories distort apperceptively any contemporary percept. The only argument that I can advance for a difference from simple projection is that we deal here with simple basic drives, which lead to simple gratifying distortions rather than to the more complex situations possible in simple projection.

Externalization

Ordinarily, a person has little awareness of the process of inverted projection, and even less of simple projection and sensitization. It is correspondingly difficult to make anyone aware of the processes in himself. On the other hand, a common experience among clinicians has the subject telling him a story about one of the TAT pictures similar to this: "This is a mother looking into the room to see if Johnny has finished his homework, and she scolds him for being tardy." On looking over the stories in the inquiry, the subject may spontaneously say, "I guess that really was the way it was with my mother and myself, though I did not realize it when I told you the story."

In psychoanalytic language one may say that this process of storytelling is preconscious; it is not conscious while it is going on but it could easily have been made so. This implies that we deal with a slightly repressed pattern of images that have an organizing effect that can be easily recalled. The term *externalization* is suggested for such a phenomenon to facilitate the clinical description of a frequently occurring process.

My teacher at Harvard, Henry Murray, has formulated a number of hypotheses concerning projection that are of particular interest here. In the first place, he chooses to differentiate between *cognitive projection* (actual misbeliefs of what he calls the Freudian type) and *imaginative projection,* which he believes is what we deal with in projective techniques. He feels that when we ask the patient to imagine something, the process involved deserves differentiation from the clinical concept of projection. Although it is a good idea to keep this in mind for distinguishing the severity of disturbance as it appears in TAT protocol, the hypothesis probably does not merit a theoretical differentiation. There are many patients who, when shown the TAT, believe that they are functioning cognitively and that their response corresponds to the actual content of the pictures. At best, one might say that the degree of ego participation or voluntary exclusion of its reality testing functions varies in the case of response to projective techniques.

However, Murray very usefully differentiates between *supplementary* projection and *complementary* projection. He reserves the first term for projection of self-constituents, that is, for the distortion of external objects by one's own needs, drives, wishes, and fears. He would speak of complementary projection as the projection of what he calls *figure-constituents,* which he defines as

> *the tendencies and qualities that characterize the figures (imaged objects) that people the subject's stream of thought and with which he interacts in fantasy. For the most part these are images of significant objects (father, mother, siblings, friends, enemies) with whom the subject has been intimately related. . . . In short, subjects are apt to ascribe self-constituents to one character (say, the hero) of the story, and figure-constituents to other characters. (Murray, 1938)*

In other words, Murray's concern centers on the definition of subtypes of projection predicated on the specific content of the projection, whereas our discussion so far has been primarily concerned with the degree of severity or complexity or relative unconsciousness of distortion. It may be profitable to combine these two points of view.

The problem of degree of distortion has also been investigated by Weisskopf. She wondered how well the TAT pictures lend themselves to projection (by eliciting more than purely cognitive perception). She developed a "transcendence index" as a quantitative measure of this factor. Subjects were instructed to describe each of the TAT pictures rather than to tell a story about it. In order to obtain the transcendence index of a picture, she counted the number of comments about the picture that went beyond pure description. The transcendence index of the picture is the mean number of such comments per subject. Pictures with high transcendence indices make impersonal observation difficult and lure the subject away from the prescribed objective path of the instructions, forcing him to project. Weisskopf found that the pictures that had high transcendence indices were those lending themselves to interpretation in terms of parent-child relationships or in terms of heterosexual relationships between contemporaries.

Pure Perception

Pure perception is the hypothetical process against which we measure apperceptive distortion of a subjective type, or it is the subjective, operationally defined agreement on the meaning of a stimulus with which other interpretations are compared. It supplies us with the end point of a continuum upon which all responses vary. Inasmuch as behavior is considered by general consent to be rational and appropriate to a given situation, we may speak of adaptive behavior to the "objective" stimulus, as discussed below.

In my own earlier experiments, I found that aggression could be induced in subjects, and that this aggression was "projected" into their stories in accordance with the projection hypothesis. I also found that under normal circumstances certain pictures are more often responded to with stories of aggression, even if the experimenter does nothing beyond simply requesting a story about the pictures. Similarly, these pictures, which by their very nature suggested aggression, lent themselves much more readily to projection of aggression than others not suggesting aggression by their content.

Of course, it seems logical that a picture showing a huddled figure and a pistol, for example, would lead to more stories of aggression than a picture of a peaceful country scene, this conclusion is nothing more than what common sense would lead one to expect. In psychological language this simply means that the response is in part a function of the stimulus. In terms of apperceptive psychology, it means that a majority of subjects agree on some basic apperception of a stimulus and that this agreement represents our operational definition of the "objective" nature of the stimulus. Behavior consistent with these "objective" reality aspects of the stimulus has been called *adaptive behavior* by G. W. Allport. If, for instance, we refer to the now-familiar card #1 of the TAT, we can say that the subjects adapt themselves to the fact that the picture shows a violin.

Several hypotheses may be formulated:

1. *The degree of adaptive behavior varies conversely with the degree of exactness of the definition of the stimulus.* TAT pictures and the Rorschach test inkblots are purposely left relatively unstructured in order to produce as many apperceptively distorted responses as possible. On the other hand, if one of the pictures of the Stanford-Binet intelligence test (e.g., the one depicting a fight between a white man and Indians) is presented, the situation is well enough defined to elicit the same response from the majority of children between the ages of 10 and 12.

2. *The exact degree of adaptation is determined also by the* Aufgabe *or set.* If the subject is asked to describe the picture, there is more adaptive behavior than if he is asked to tell a story about it. In the latter case he tends to disregard many objective aspects of the stimulus. For instance, suppose an air-raid siren is sounded. The behavior of the subject who expects to hear sirens and knows what to do when he hears them will differ greatly from the behavior of the subject who does not know the significance of the sound. To the latter, the noise might mean anything from a work stoppage to a catastrophe.

3. *The nature of the perceiving organism also determines the ratio of adaptive versus projective behavior,* as previously discussed. For example, a person's reaction to a stimulus when he is awake may be entirely different from his reaction when he is awakened by the same stimulus.

Expressive behavior is different from both adaptation and apperceptive distortion. Given a fixed ratio of adaptation and apperceptive distortion in a subject's response to either Stanford-Binet picture, individuals may still vary in their style and in their organization. One might use long sentences with many adjectives; another might use short sentences with pregnant phrases of strictly logical sequence. If individuals write their responses, they may vary as to upper and lower length in spacing. If they speak, they may differ in speed, pitch, or volume. All these are personal characteristics that are fairly stable for every person. Similarly, the artist may chisel in small detail with precision or choose a less exacting form. He may arrange things either symmetrically or off center. And again, in response to the air-raid signal, a person may run, crouch, jump, walk, or talk—and do each of these things in his own typical way.

In a similar way, expressive behavior influences the TAT productions, accounting for individual differences in style, sentence structure, verb-noun ratio, and other formal characteristics. Expressive features reveal, then, how one does something; adaptation and apperceptive distortion concern what one does. If this is the case, it is needless to emphasize that one can always ask how one does what one does. *Adaptive, apperceptive, and expressive behavior are always coexistent.*

A Restatement of the Metapsychology of Projecting: Apperceiving as a Variant of Perception

The adaptive features of the apperceptive process have long been underestimated not only by clinicians but also by academic psychologists until they discovered the effects of motivation on perception. Clinicians have been aware of the fact that there is always a kernel of truth even in paranoid delusions, but have concerned themselves primarily with the distorted factors.

The matter of "style," of how one does what one does, seems relevant to psychological testing, artistic creativity, and many forms of behavior. This aspect of cognition, called *cognitive style,* was given particular prominence by the work of Holzman and Klein and others, who spoke of "levelers" and "sharpeners." The concept relates to the degree with which persons merge new experiences with memories of earlier experiences. These memories may be either conscious or unconscious, and become either increasingly bolder in relief or "level out."

The concept of leveling is particularly important for a

general discussion of the process of defense mechanisms. Obviously, an extreme of leveling relates not only to repression but to apperceptive distortion of any experience by the previously acquired apperceptive mass. It is likely that leveling is related primarily to the normally present and necessary synthesizing function of the ego. This function, when absent, can account in part for dissociative phenomena; when excessive, it can account for pathological repression. A relationship of leveling and sharpening to the synthesizing function would make more reasonable the authors' assumption that leveling-sharpening is an enduring aspect of ego organization. (I consider the synthetic functions to be often mostly congenitally determined.) Selective leveling and sharpening of various composites of one stimulus may play a role in reaction formation, where the acceptable features are sharpened and the unacceptable ones leveled.

The structural aspects of apperception can probably be stated most succinctly by paraphrasing Eissler, who said that *perception becomes structure*. One might add that, in turn, structure influences perception. Even as Eissler said that continuing perceptual experiences become the structure of the personality, we may emphasize that the past apperceptive mass continually influences contemporary perception. Aside from the other experiential data, structural aspects of the ego apparatus that might have to be labeled as autonomous also affect apperception, as do intelligence, the synthetic function of the ego, and the various *Anlagen* (predispositions), presumably constituting a biological, constitutional, and heredity precursor of the later ego.

In this context, we could define *projection* as an extreme of apperceptive distortion where the previous apperceptive mass, or certain aspects of the previous apperceptive mass, has so much of a controlling effect on contemporary perception that it seriously impairs the adaptive aspects of cognition. In other words, the primary process "contaminates" the secondary process.

The relative predominance of primary and secondary

process can be thought of as on a continuum in a variety of psychological processes. In a dream there is a predominance of apperceptive mass and a relative minimum of ego functioning; in hypnotic phenomena, the self-observing functions and other cognitive forces of the ego are decreased (as in the process of falling asleep), but at the same time they are structured by some motivational force. Similarly, in a preconscious fantasy, the apperceptive mass has a greater influence than the adaptive cognition; however, since this process is preconscious, it is easily reversed so that adaptive, cognitive functions take over. *Déjà vu* phenomena and depersonalization, the response to projective techniques, and the process of free association need to be placed in this continuum of relative predominance of apperceptive mass over adaptive functioning, and the role of repression in the service of certain adaptive functions of the ego.

The genetic aspect of apperception and its extreme variant, the process of projecting, are intimately related to the nucleus of all psychological theory. The consensus today is probably that we do not start out as a *tabula rasa* but rather with a set of *Anlagen* and precursors of the ego apparatus as well as drive characteristics.

The hypothesis that all apperception is structured by some previous, once-upon-a-time apperception, leaves the problem of the first apperception. Of course I believe that, in terms of *gestalt* theory, there is at first little differentiation of figure and ground, and that articulation of percepts and various hierarchical relationships between experiences are only slowly established. The concept of the primary process and the slow emergence of the secondary process are the analytic processes relating to this area of psychology.

In attempting to construct genetic models of projecting, the idea of "spitting out" of noxious or unpleasant stimuli has been used. By this token, too, projection has been said to have a certain oral basis. A similar notion plays a role in Melanie Klein's formulations of projections of the "good breast" and the "bad breast." These formulations seem to have some explanatory value in certain childhood ideas of fear of poisoning, probably also related to anal concepts (dirty, sexual material ingested does harm and may be ejected either orally or anally). Perception, however, also needs to be considered in its broadest perspective—of individuation of the differential perception of the self and others. It is on this level that projection and depersonalization must be seen as interrelated concepts. The oral, genetic concept needs supplementation by visual, thermal, tactile, proprioceptive, and other perceptual cues related to the development of the self-concept and later interactions between self and nonself.

The qualities of the unconscious thought processes can probably be best understood in terms of the genesis of the apperceptive mass. When we speak of transference phenomena, I think of the apperceptive distortion of the contemporary figure of the analyst by (to use Murray's terms) self-constituents or figure constituents of the past: The analyst becomes the object of oral, masochistic, phallic, or other demands and may be experienced as if he were father, mother, or whatever. In understanding the transference distortions and in attaining insight and working through apperceptive distortions, we try in essence to isolate various genetic components of the contemporary apperception. The clinically present *gestalt* or configuration has to be "analyzed" into its component parts.

As all current apperception is viewed through something like a composite of all experiential data, we find that no contemporary apperception has a one-to-one relationship to a specific experience of the past, but is constantly impressed by overdetermination of each experience. Dream imagery, of course, gives the most vivid account of the contamination of contemporary experience by many layers of past images.

The topographical aspects of apperception have been briefly touched on earlier. If the process ranges from adaptive behavior to sensitization, externalization, simple projection, and inverted projection, it obviously ranges from conscious to preconscious to unconscious spheres of activity.

The strictly economic aspects of apperception are

clearly important if one remembers that object-cathexis is largely a matter of cathexis of internalized objects, and that indeed the increase or decrease of stimulus value is largely affected by the apperceptive mass.

The problems of the dynamics of apperception are of immediate interest. They are related to the entire concept of defense mechanisms. (Academic psychologists have in part approached the problem by speaking of "perceptual defense.") Yet the clinician reading my restatement of many psychoanalytic concepts within the perceptual and apperceptive framework may find himself with the nagging question: "So what?" He may acknowledge the potential scientific interest of the exercise, yet wonder if it has any significance for the store of working concepts he uses daily. In the next and final section, I shall review some of these.

Perception and Clinical Phenomena

Perceptive and apperceptive restatements can be offered for common clinical constructs, such as ego strength, defenses, and mechanisms of dream work, as well as for concrete clinical instances.

Ego Strength

In Chapter Six, I discuss in detail my conceptualization of the ego and methods for measuring and evaluating its functioning. For now, I will limit the discussion to perception's relevance to the concept of "ego strength" as it is used in everyday clinical work.

Many phenomena of ego weakness can be primarily characterized by perceptual disturbance, specifically a disturbance of the differentiation of past apperceptions from contemporary ones. For instance, in the normal weakening of ego strength associated with falling asleep, we speak of hypnagogic phenomena. There, the apperception of reality is distorted by the memory traces of past apperceptions.

Indeed, dreams themselves may be understood in these terms, as will be discussed later in this section.

Ordinarily, the clinical diagnosis of conditions characterized by extreme ego disturbance (i.e., ego weakness) is primarily made by observing phenomenological characteristics. Clinically, phenomena of unreality and evidence of the primary process in apperception are evidence of structural weakness—the lack of clear definition of the apperceptions disturbed by the past.

The characteristic of ego strength, in terms of apperceptive clarity, is comparable to physical structures. A middling amount of stability is desirable. If there is too little fixedness, support is lacking; with too much fixedness, structures are brittle. The rigid apperceptive constitution of the obsessive compulsive sacrifices adaptability for the sake of some stability. The firmness of organization of images may be overdone. And, of course, alcohol and other anesthetics may loosen the arrangement and weaken the ego through their effect on brain function.

Defenses

The defenses were originally entirely anthropomorphized concepts, particularly the concept of the "censor" responsible for repression in dreams. Defenses can probably be entirely conceptualized, however, in terms of apperception. Repression, as the most basic form of defense, is truly inherent in the entire concept of unconsciousness. For example, the fact that some characteristics of mother or some memories of her behavior are "repressed" is part of the construction of the composite photograph.

The idea of "defense" has a perfectly good correlative in the buffer systems of the bodily organism, namely, the alkali reserve. Cannon's concept of homeostasis had its early forerunner in Freud's thinking and is now freely used by psychoanalysts. It is probably consistent with the perceptual principles of the tendency toward the "good" *gestalt* (Prägnanz), which on the other hand finds its equivalent in the formation of crystals and the formation of globules in fluid in such a way that the most stable form is the one where all forces are "equalized." In other words, the psychoanalytic concepts of defense can probably be understood as a tendency to achieve the most stable system, or to permit minimum disturbance of an established system of forces in an apperception. The latter embodies the concept of the ego as a barrier to excessive external or internal stimulation.

One may also state it this way: Defense mechanisms can be considered the selective and structuring effect of certain image properties on the effect of past apperceptions on present apperceptions. Each separate defense mechanism formulated by psychoanalysis constitutes a hypothesis concerning some lawfulness of interaction of images under certain circumstances.

The mechanism of denial, for example, can most easily be understood as the apperception of a contemporary situation in a way least likely to upset a (precarious) apperceptive balance. When a mother has aggressive and affectionate feelings for her child at the same time, one of the possible results of this conflict of sentiments is described by psychoanalysis as reaction formation. The aggressive feelings are repressed and become unconscious, and only excessive affection is manifest.

Dreams

Freud often spoke with affection of what he called his dream book, and many analysts especially enjoy dream interpretation. Many of the basic processes involved can be understood in perceptual terms. In the dream book, Freud spoke of condensation, secondary elaboration, and symbolization.

Dreams often appear to be a chaotic jumble. This is partly because perceptions from different times are coalesced (the "transparencies" I mentioned in the last section). Thus a grotesque dream figure may actually consist of features of different people or animals; and it takes free association to trace it back to the elements, or partial *gestalten,* which have now achieved closure in this particularly nightmarish image.

Condensation

The process of greatest utility for understanding in *gestalt* perceptual terms is that of condensation. Condensation can be understood as a new closure or new *gestalt* formation. The dream figures may sometimes seem nonsensical because of this process of combining different *gestalten* to form a new one. Of course this also holds true for psychotic productions, such as hallucinations. Seen in these terms, however, it becomes obvious that creative processes such as painting, creative writing, and other expressions result from the new *gestalt* formation.

Secondary Elaboration

When a dreamer reports a dream, he is understood to elaborate, adding to the dream as it occurred. He makes connections between what appear originally as meaningless pieces, a process best understood as "closure." For instance, one looks at a Picasso single-line drawing with much interrupted space, but nevertheless perceives it as a whole figure through the process of closure.

Symbolization

The dream, by virtue of the *gestalt* formation it involves, contains perceptions from many different phases of a patient's life. Specifically, it is held that the dream will contain (1) the "day residue" or perceptual material that comes from the last 24 hours, and constitutes the patient's attempt at coping and thinking in the dream; (2) the transference situation (if the patient is in treatment); and finally (3) the material from any part of the patient's life history, selected for its relationship to the day residue. Once more, the analytic job is to "analyze" or to dissolve the final complex and unintelligible *gestalt* of the manifest dream into the parts that constitute what it symbolizes. The value of perceiving dreams in the terms of perceptual theory, however, is generally not recognized by psychoanalysts or academic psychologists.

Free Association

For free associating, it is necessary to permit a poor definition of the contemporary apperception, precisely so that past images may emerge. In what I have called the "oscillating function" of the ego, it is at the same time necessary to compare the past apperception with the contemporary apperception, and observe differences.

Let me now illustrate my view with a few specific clinical examples. Many therapists have heard a version of the frequent dream in which the dreamer struggles up some steps that seem to be almost as high as he, and most likely scare him. What is occurring in such a case is most likely that an earlier life experience of the child climbing up steps has now translated itself into an adult dream of the difficulty of taking steps. Many of the steps in these dreams may have a distinctive characteristic, and usually the patient can go back to the precise origin of this *gestalt*. The dream is easier to understand by locating it in time and by associating it with a person, in this case the person in whose house the child originally saw the steps.

In clinical practice, transference distortion, which is a highly individualized perception of the therapist's face and personality, is frequent. In the first session, before initiating therapy, I will often ask patients what they dreamed the night before the initial session. Some will have had a dream of a mad scientist chasing them with a long syringe, whereas others will have dreamed that they were being treated to a lavish and sumptuous meal. Clearly, the first patient expects me to be a pretty harmful fellow, whereas the second patient expects to come to therapy and be lovingly nurtured.

Sometimes the same material that appears in dreams can appear in psychotic experiences. One patient, when she was psychotic, believed she was surrounded by a group of 12 cats sitting around a table in judgment of her. When she recompensated, the same images were in her dreams.

The origin of such phenomena can be seen in another disturbed patient. One young psychotic man on the ward had been admitted because he feared some people were trying to kill him. In taking the man's history, it appeared that as a child he had nightmares of being attacked by antediluvian animals. Later, in adult life, he continued to have dreams of this nature. By describing a few characteristics, it was easy to identify the dinosaurs as parental figures, whom he feared and viewed as sadistic, with good reason—his parents had often beat him in childhood.

In another case (mentioned in Chapter Two), the patient had repeated nightmares of being attacked by the Viet Cong, which were clearly related to childhood dreams of being pursued by a gorilla. By a few signs, such as a particular hat the animal wore, it was easy to identify the gorilla as a threatening, punitive mother and understand the influence of these early perceptions on the man's later perception of the Viet Cong.

Object Relations Theory

Object relations theories, in all their variations, are basically perceptual. Melanie Klein, who formulated the concept of the bad breast as an infantile perception, believed this tended to structure perceptions of people throughout their lives. Winnicott, Kernberg, and Mahler all speak of the acquisition of percepts—the self and objects and their influence on each other. They all fail to avail themselves of the advantage of stating their theory in terms of *gestalt* theory generally, and the acquisition of percepts specifically. Their divergent views can best be understood as different notions of the acquisition and interaction of percepts; yet percepts of the self and objects—and part-object and self-object interactions—could benefit vastly from discussion in the perceptual terms of *gestalt* theory and the concept of apperception discussed earlier. *Gestalten* perceptions become structure and, as such, continue to govern the nature of lifelong perceptions.

CHAPTER FOUR

Psychoanalysis as a Trait Psychology

Introduction

One of the most striking changes to occur in academic psychology during my time is the change in interest of the study of personality understood as a trait psychology. The psychologist graduating today has probably encountered traits in one of two ways. He may have studied not the traits themselves but the information processing involved in perceiving or thinking about traits. In that case, the study is really about the perceiver or the thinker, not the person whose traits are being perceived or thought about. Or he may have encountered traits in a history and systems class, or some advanced seminar on theory development.

From the earliest days of interest in traits, the concept has been something of an amphibian term, partly a creature of common sense and partly a creature of the science of psychology.

The *Oxford English Dictionary* defines a *trait* as a particular feature of the mind or character and cites uses of this sense of the word dating from the mid-eighteenth century. Understood as an ordinary word, and not as a technical term that implies something static, there could have been (and, I believe, should be) an emphasis on some natural affinities between psychoanalysis and trait theory. The ordinary term, after all, says nothing about how a trait developed, what dynamic or economic functions it performs, or any of the other questions that psychoanalysis attempts to answer. Later in this chapter, I will make some of these connections explicit.

The history of science, however, is a continuing process in which the entry of scientific methods forces out or modifies ordinary understandings. Classification—making taxonomies—is the start of many sciences. The botanist who lands on an island makes endless lists, trying to group together variations into types; the concept of trait can be seen as an effort to follow this practice.

You are probably familiar with many systems and types. Carl Jung contrasted the outgoing extravert with the inward-looking introvert. Sheldon (1954) classified according to body build: the short, plump endomorph was sociable, relaxed, and even tempered; the tall, thin ectomorph was restrained and solitary; and the muscular mesomorph was noisy, active, and sometimes coarse.

Hans Eysenck, a critic of psychoanalysis who will be discussed at greater length in Chapter Eight, developed a well-known classificatory system that uses the trait pairs stable-unstable and introverted-extraverted as dimensions that intersect one another, so that a given individual can be located in a two-dimensional Cartesian space.

Historically, classifications have been made in many ways. Inventories have been taken, which ask the subject to answer questions about situations. The answers are then translated into profiles or scores. For example, if you say that you enjoy speaking up in meetings, this answer would, on the face of it, suggest extraversion. Some inventories use questions where the meaning of the answer is not obvious, so that many questions are given to large groups and distinctive answer patterns are identified. For example, there is no reason to think that a schizophrenic person would necessarily say "yes" if asked whether the color red was like a bell; yet it might turn out that this is the case, and would allow the psychologist to use the question later when classifying others. Of course, these approaches assume a certain level of cooperation, which is sometimes lacking.

While the development of these research tools goes beyond common sense in allowing quantification and multidimensional classification, the scientist may find himself unhappy unless he is able to elaborate. In particular, trait approaches have been criticized for dealing with characteristics in isolation and for failing to describe functional relations among traits.

To some degree, psychoanalysts may claim credit for the declining interest in traits, and they may have to share the blame. Given that there is a rather fundamental tension between the dynamic emphasis of psychoanalysis and the more static conceptions of trait psychology, the increasing influence of psychoanalysis after World War II may have pushed out (and partly usurped) a portion of the interest in trait psychology. However, I shall argue in this chapter that the existence of this very real tension between the two approaches does not rule out some *rapprochement*. I shall also offer a psychoanalytically based way of understanding traits, which retains some of the original meaning but introduces a more dynamic conceptualization.

Traits

Although trait theory once enjoyed more prestige (especially in Europe) than it does today, scientific psychologists, especially in the United States, have a long history of distrusting trait theory. I imagine that it is too close for comfort to the commonsense psychology of the man in the street, who quite regularly explains behavior as an expression of or as caused by a personality trait. And if the scientific psychologists cannot see themselves as knowing more than the man in the street, they will wonder why they wasted so much time in graduate school and why anyone would pay them for specialist knowledge. Thus there has been a natural tendency for focused, strictly defined scientific aspirations to be negatively correlated with sympathy for trait theory, leaving trait theory to be represented by psychologists with more wide-ranging definitions of their subject matter.

The most prominent examples may be the work of a brilliant British polymath psychologist who came to Duke University in North Carolina, William McDougall, and my teacher at Harvard, G. W. Allport.

McDougall indeed ranged widely, publishing studies of the brain, applying experimental methods to the study of the psychology of the people of Borneo, and, as his career progressed, moving steadily in the direction of the larger formations of the psyche (e.g., sentiments, attitudes, personalities, etc.). Probably he was most known for his book *Social Psychology*. The idea for the book occurred to him in 1906, when he was lecturing: He wondered if the energy visible in every human activity might be some complex but definite product of an inborn disposition or instinct.

G. W. Allport drew on many European theorists now popular among those who take the so-called hermeneutical (i.e., interpretive) approach to psychology. Allport developed a theory of personality that introduced functional descriptions, and drew on interpretive approaches to envision the overall integration of trait characteristics, so that they were not viewed in isolation.

Psychoanalysis and Traits

I believe that there can be useful interaction between trait theory and psychoanalysis. The former can help establish links between psychodynamic formulations on the one hand, and common sense and classificatory approaches on the other. The latter can add dynamics and can provide a more fully explanatory approach that tackles functional and economic questions. The most effective way to make the needed translation is via the theory of libidinal development. I will review this theory in the sections that follow, and then close the chapter by drawing some connections between psychoanalytic work and trait theory.

What I have called a "translation" between trait theory and psychoanalysis is in reality a further specification. In what follows, trait theory is enriched developmentally and by reference to specifiable physiological structures and their functioning; psychoanalysis is enriched, by emphasis rather than revision, by bringing into focus the overlap between libidinal aims and organizing personality characteristics.

Libidinal Development

Psychoanalysis attempts to relate the "types" it discusses to the body, not just in a classificatory way (as with Sheldon's body builds, discussed earlier), but as a way of understanding how the development of a type has its origins in features of physical development and functioning.

The earliest stage of libidinal investment is conceived of as a diffuse cathexis of the whole body. This is increasingly focused (in a way that has not yet been specified) into a greater specific hedonic tone of the oral zone, to be followed and overlapped by the anal area. This is followed by and superimposed at the end of infancy onto the phallic stage as the early aspect of focusing on a genital zone, to be interrupted by the latency period and to be matured into the genital zone proper as the preferred zone of pleasure seeking with the end of puberty. These propositions can be stated as an orderly maturational sequence of preferred loci of stimulation. Even as such, the propositions still need clear-cut observational verification and more specific statement.

Experiments would have to be devised in which standard oral, anal, and genital stimulation are provided at given intervals during the years of childhood, and some criteria are chosen for determining the preference. Aside from the fact that such experiments should certainly not be detrimental to a subject's development, it is not easy to think of the proper experimental design. Recording of infants' reaction to standard stimuli is, however, by no means a new or difficult idea, as I discuss in Chapter Four.

Libidinal Aims

Aside from defining the somatic areas that are preferred as foci of gratification, the libido theory includes statements concerning the nature of the operations involved in gratification of libidinal aims at various stages of development. These are also spoken of as partial or component sexual aims, since they may be part or components of later genital activity. Thus the theory of libidinal aims is a set of propositions concerned with the sequence, interaction, and fate of preferences for gratifying operations throughout life. These operations may be in part a function of maturational processes of the endocrine-nervous system, and in part related to learned stimulus-response patterns. If we borrow a phrase from the brain psychologist Lashley, we might think of these aims as perceptual choices in response to deficit states. *Perceptual choices* and *stimulus response* should not be understood in primitive conditioned reflex terms but rather in the form of complex interactions of configurations *(gestalten),* as will be discussed below.

1. Corresponding to the earliest undifferentiated zone (which for classification purposes is included in the oral phase, since the relationship between feeding and skin sensation at the mother's breast has been shown) are undifferentiated aims of skin stimulation, rhythmic muscular activity, and splanchnic gratification, already related to the oral phase's aim of sucking.

2. More specifically, the oral aims are subdivided into the passive (sucking) subphase and the active oral (incorporating, biting) subphase.

3. The anal phase is subdivided into the aim to retain and the aim to expel (aggressively). Sadistic-masochistic aims are considered characterologic derivatives of this phase.

4. The early genital or phallic phase, including urethral phase, was added by Freud to his pregenital and genital conceptions with these words:

> *I later (1925) altered this in that I interpolated a third phase into the development of the child after the two pregenital organizations, one which indeed deserves the name of a genital, one which reveals a sexual object and a measure of convergence of the sexual strivings upon this object, but which differs in one essential point from the definitive organization of sexual maturity. That is, it knows only one sort of genital, the male. I have therefore called it the phallic stage of organization. (Freud, 1905)*

(The clitoris may play the role of the phallic organ for the girl.) Its biological prototype, according to Abraham, is the homogeneous genital *Anlage* of the embryo undifferentiated for either sex.

The basic assumption of the phallic phase of libidinal development is that the aim and modes of gratification are now focused on the penis and its female biological equivalent, the clitoris. (Clinically, there are many forms of an illusory phallus [e.g., fecal]; and adult female patients often seem to conceive of the cervix as an indwelling phallus.) The implication for object relations is that in contrast to the autoerotic pregenital phase, phallic gratification is desired from an external object, originally from one specific object.

In Chapter Two, I concentrate on aspects of psychoanalysis that can be well understood as theories of learning. From the standpoint of learning, the phallic phase may be of particular importance for the development of a girl. If the little girl has a brother who is greatly favored, she may feel that it would be better to be a boy and she may become "fixated" at the phallic level. Not only is she a tomboy as a child but she stays identified with masculine activities, viewpoints, and aims into adulthood. She may possibly be overassertively denying the lack of a phallus, she may be particularly aggressive toward males whom she envies the phallus and wants to "castrate," or she may make male object-choices (of boyfriends, husbands) who have a large feminine component.

Other learning experiences may also fixate a girl at the phallic phase of gratification. (The term *condition* or *fixate by conditioning* could be substituted for this usage of *fixate*.) If the role of the mother is a particularly suffering one (e.g., at the hands of a sadistic husband); if the child is particularly exposed to parental intercourse (primal scene) or has particularly realistic reasons for a sadistic conception of things done to the mother; or if the situation is so structured that the child becomes particularly aware of menstrual bleeding and connects this with ideas of genital traumatization of the female—all these learning experiences may tend to arrest her at the level of attempting to maintain that she is a boy rather than a girl.

The urethral phase is sometimes treated as an independent intermediary stage between the pregenital and the phallic, and sometimes as part of the phallic. The latter designation seems more appropriate, both clinically and logically.

The urethral phase is usually conceived of as twofold: the active form, accompanied by fantasies of penetration and exhibitionism, and the more passive form of "letting flow." The latter is clinically often seen related to the oral phase (e.g., in cases of premature ejaculation in which the patient reports a pleasant feeling of the penis being enveloped by the vaginal walls "like a body being embraced," and other associations further relating to being fed and loved by the mother). Ejaculation in such cases frequently takes place from an unerect penis and without a feeling of climax, the patient reporting that "it really was more like urinating."

In more detail, the aims of the urethral phase of gratification are not only that of urinating but often urinating competitively—seeing who can aim higher—and wanting to be admired for one's prowess. To be sure, the intermediary position of the phallic phase is also borne out by the fact that some of the urinary pleasures may be more of an autoerotic nature, while others are definitely object-related. On the other hand, more definitely phallic connotations appear in the fact that some little girls want to "urinate like boys," standing up, and by this activity stake their claims to phallic.

Learning propositions enter in where, for instance, the child is submitted early to severe urinary training, or where there is general overemphasis on urinary functions. Again, frequent occasions for comparison with an older male, or reasons for excessive masculine identification in a female child (e.g., in a strong homosexual relation to a sister) may reinforce urethral aims to a point where they predominate in character formation or in the creation of neurotic syndromes.

Characterologically, the psychoanalytic proposition is that urethral aims will later manifest themselves in the wish to be looked at (exhibitionism) and to look (voyeurism [e.g., for comparison of genitals]). If such aims are sublimated, a career such as acting on the stage or examining as a microbiologist, may be a result. More diffusely, a urethral character would be one who is very ambitious, competitive, and show-offish.

The degree to which this aim is expressed in behavior depends on how early the urethral aim was strengthened by the mother's conditioning and other environmental circumstances. That is, if the urethral aim is excessive, it is considered apt to produce pathological manifestations (from perversions to premature ejaculation, to character disorders, to sublimated character traits). However, as with other statements concerning libidinal propositions, we should state here that these propositions are made appropriately much more complex by other propositions: The isolated event of increased urethral aims must be seen in the total pattern of the personality. Similarly, other statements concerning libido theory have to be qualified. For instance, even if a mother should particularly stress urethral performance but should otherwise afford the child a "healthy" psychological climate, the urethral problem might appear only in a sublimated or at least nondisturbing pathological form (e.g., a [voyeuristic] hobby in an otherwise well-functioning person such as collecting opera glasses), while the same maternal behavior in an otherwise pathogenic environment might lead to a specific urethrogenic psychopathology; while again, in a third environment of extreme pathogenicity, a schizophrenic picture might be produced in which the urethral pathology is the least of the patient's troubles.

5. The latency period is one of the more embattled psychoanalytic concepts. This is mostly because Freud originally related it to phylogenetic influences. Nearly all psychoanalysts have given up this speculation and hold that ontogenetic propositions adequately explain its existence. Another point of contention has concerned its lawful appearance. There are those who maintain it reflects ontogenetic maturational processes, and those who maintain that the latency period is strictly the result of (cultural) learning.

Stated simply, the proposition concerning aims of gratification in the latency period (roughly from the fifth to the tenth year) means that there is an inhibition of direct pregenital or phallic aims (i.e., these aims are not observed or are observed less than before and after this period). Instead, what is observed and is presumed to be causally related to the erstwhile manifest phallic aims (now inhibited by the superego) are sublimations of this aim, manifesting themselves in *intellectual* curiosity. The infantile aims are also sublimated in part, and in part reaction formations take place. The ego is strengthened, possibly by a maturational ebbing of active striving and resultant better control, and also by the emergence of the superego (out of the resolution of the oedipus complex).

Thus a concept of the "latency period" involves at least the following:

> a. The assumption, postulation, or demonstration of a biological, endocrine, maturational process characterized by a decrease in a sexual drive (in all its psychoanalytic submeanings).
> b. A strengthening of the ego, partly secondary to the weakening of the id drives and partly due

to the perceptual, motor, and intellectual growth of the ego (a strengthening of the "autonomous functions" as Hartmann calls them). The secondary strengthening of the ego is itself predicated on a set of propositions; namely, that it is part of the ego's functions to mediate between drive demand and reality, and to exercise control generally, and that such control is "easier" when the drive demand is decreased. The further proposition involved is that if the ego can "spare some energy" from controlling the id, it can use this energy for other tasks (e.g., sublimating the drive).

c. The concept of sublimation: Drives may change their mode of gratification, their aim, from direct gratification to some detour behavior that is more consistent with the entire set of cultural demands and maturational change. For example, the wish to look at someone's genitals may be generalized into curiosity concerning the nature of the universe and learning generally, toward mastery of the environment.

6. Adolescent-adult genitality phase is ordinarily associated with sexuality, that there eventually will be a union of the genitals in copulation. It is important in the concept of adult genital aims that psychoanalysis recognizes all preceding pregenital and early genital aims as appropriate components of the genital aim *per se,* provided the components play a secondary role and terminate in the genital union. Perversion, psychoanalytically, exists where any component pregenital aim supersedes the genital aim. This definition is of course psychological, not sociological or normative, and should not be considered a judgment.

Ego, Id, and Superego

The elements of the so-called structural theory are not, strictly speaking, traits. I will say more about my conceptualizations in Chapter Six, but for now I can state that they provide a mode by which various libidinal aims exert and influence abiding configurational aspects of personality.

The Ego

A new era in psychoanalysis began when attention turned to analysis not only of the unconscious but also of the ego and its defenses. This swing of the pendulum allowed for a larger scope for trait conceptualization. It also increased the recognizability of some of the concepts. For instance, who but a psychoanalyst would consider speaking of his well-respected neighbor, who is a fireman, as demonstrating traits of urethral exhibitionism? By the time something is recognizably a trait, it has undergone the influence of ego structures and appears in "tamer" form. Historically, too, study of the ego has been more socially acceptable; perhaps this fact may have allowed for more overlap with common sense and academic psychological concepts, such as traits.

Theoretical assumptions concerning the ego are twofold, based on both constitutional, genetic maturational processes and on principles of learning. Even though Freud stated quite clearly that there is no reason why there should not be primary, congenital ego variations, it was only in the 1950s that these two basic assumptions were made somewhat overt (e.g., in Hartmann's work).

Enlightened behavioral science—especially American—is often reluctant to consider the significance of genetic and congenital factors; this is partly a reaction to earlier overemphasis on genetics and partly an aspect of our cultural era. Birth and heredity were so all-determining in past centuries that the Declaration of Independence found it necessary to proclaim that "all men are created equal." Much of the sentiment in American psychology against the genetic orientation of psychoanalysis, its determinism and biological orientation, is influenced by these cultural trends. These are precisely the factors responsible for some of the antagonism to McDougall's work on traits (mentioned earlier).

The ego can best be described by its history, by its functions, and, most importantly, by the extent to which it fulfills its functions in a quantitative way. Spitz has probably stated most clearly the perspective on historical events. His 1959 theory of ego development outlines a series of hypothesized stages, each marked by specific affective behavior, and involving so-called "organizers of the psyche," which integrate maturational and psychological developmental factors. At three months, the first organizer, the smiling response, manifests itself as the beginning of the ego and also of structural perception and reality testing. The second organizer (at eight months) is a tendency to show distress in the presence of strangers, indicating recognition of the mother and heralding "attainment of the libidinal object." This demonstration of memory and judgment, as well as some understanding of social gestures and the emergence of some defenses, thus coincides with the development of major ego functions. Spitz's third organizer, the attainment of the No, demonstrates that the ego has developed the capacity for abstraction and reversibility. These "concepts of dependent development, critical periods, and the synchronicity of maturation and development" lead Spitz to conclude that a deficiency in maturational or psychological development occurs, and "a deviant integration will result, which creates a developmental imbalance" and therefore unbalances other ego-related and developmental structures (Bellak, Hurvich, & Gediman, 1973).

There is observational evidence, and it seems likely on neurological and general development grounds (Melanie Klein's view notwithstanding), that there is little differentiation of psychic function in the infant prior to the sixth month. At first the infant probably has poorly defined sensory impressions, without differentiation of his own body from the rest of the world or differentiation of his proprioceptive and other subjective perceptions from reality *per se*. In fact, observational and experimental evidence shows that body and mind are one, in the sense that perceptual stimulation seems necessary for somatic development.

In Chapter Three, I focus on the perceptual theory involved in my view of psychoanalysis. Let me here confine the argument to understanding how libidinal aims and ego structures can affect expressive qualities in perception. This idea is not an unfamiliar one; consider the commonplace that the bitter man sees the world as filled with disappointments, whereas the happy man sees it as filled with opportunities.

Only when perceptions become clearly differentiated into figure and ground—at least so that the child can differentiate the surface of his own body from the rest of the world—can the child be expected to tell the difference between subjective and objective phenomena. It is then presumably that one may speak of an ego, as Freud did in *The Ego and the Id* (1923): "The ego is first and foremost a body ego; it is not merely a surface entity but it is itself the projection of a surface."

Thus, starting with the perception of the body as figure and the rest of the world as ground, psychoanalysis refers to the ego as that aspect of mental functioning concerned with (1) the ordering of reality into figure and ground and (2) the awareness of this and other intricate relationships between apperceptions and their memory. In the most severe disturbances of the mental functioning, the psychoses, this differentiation of body and the rest of the world in part breaks down again.

It is consistent with the psychoanalytic theory that all structured mentation starts with perception. The ego comprises those apperceptions that are conscious or can easily become conscious. It also includes those that are continuously part of the contemporary apperceptions in a way that permits one to differentiate (by experience) various figure and ground judgments (e.g., external versus internal. One can then exercise "good judgment" founded on past experience (memory traces of past apperceptions) as to what is safe and what is not, what is probable and what is not. In this context, there can be no doubt that intelligence enters in as the ability to form new "wholes" out of old "parts" and to find solutions to new problems never encountered in that form. In that sense, intelligence truly becomes an organizing function.

The ego is said to have executive functions concerning the motor system. Presumably they are related to the early apperception of kinesthetic stimuli and their differentiation from external and other stimuli, and the reactivation of kinesthetic memory images in the process of bodily manipulation.

Thinking, considered by Freud a form of trial action, can at least in part be conceptualized as the recall of past apperceptions—visual, auditory, and so on. Problem solving presumably occurs by closure concerning past apperceptions and the contemporary apperceptions of the "problem." Intuition, so long a matter of speculation, probably refers to the fact that a new configuration may arise as more than just the sum of the parts that went into it, or else without conscious awareness of the process of restructuration or even of the parts that went into it. In the same way, any visual stimulus may be apperceived as a whole without conscious awareness of the parts that make up the total picture.

Into the ego's development go many learning experiences, inasmuch as the reality that is tested differs greatly in different cultures. In fact, even the degree of differentiation of contemporary apperception from past apperception, and of subjective and objective varies from culture to culture. Probably people without psychosis could have hallucinations in other cultures, since what may be socially acceptable behavior in one culture has to be rejected by the ego as unacceptable by another culture.

The Id

Much could be said about the id, but I will confine myself to a couple of remarks relevant to trait considerations. The id was Freud's term, borrowed from Groddeck (1923), which originally stood for all that was felt as ego alien—"it makes me feel like crying." Freud himself has suggested that the term may originally go back to Nietzsche. Conceptually speaking, the id became the hypothetical locus and mainspring of the drives; covertly, the psychoanalytic concept of the id is part of the psychoanalytic theory of motivation. It is not, however, the entire theory of motivation, as some would mistakenly have it, since psychoanalysis deals very complexly with a motivational system that takes into account not only the complex assumptions concerning drives (as already discussed in part as the libido theory) but also their genetic and dynamic and economic interaction with each other, with the superego, the ego, and the environment.

The concept of the id primarily implies the assumption of primary organismic drives. Psychoanalysis then formulates specific hypotheses concerning maturational changes of these drives, and the impact of environmental learning upon them and interaction with them. As far as the primary drives are concerned we can safely expect biologists, experimental psychologists and neurologists to advance the soundest hypotheses, which should then lend themselves to the additional specific hypothesis that psychoanalysts know best.

Again, psychoanalysis has made a few formal statements of a principle often implied, namely that there are probably congenital id variations, primarily in the strength of the drives. Thus one person's ego may be predestined for a more difficult time simply because this particular person starts out life with a more vigorous id than another person. This may be partly responsible for the common observation of variation in the overall energy level among different personalities.

The Superego

The superego is the structural concept of psychoanalysis concerned with "moral" behavior, insofar as this moral behavior is based on unconscious, early learned behavioral patterns. Alexander's suggestion to speak of conscience in distinction from superego when we speak of conscious, ego-syntonic precepts of social behavior is probably a widely accepted one.

There are analysts who maintain that the superego also has genetic, constitutional aspects aside from what we could readily identify as learned components. This idea seems difficult to accept unless it be made part of a broader concept; namely, that some organisms seem to have less drive demand than others and that this is not primarily a function of lack of drive but—if such a distinction can be made—of excess of control. The difficulty lies in the assumption that "moral control" would be constituted separately from those control factors usually identified with the ego.

From a learning standpoint, the superego is the totality of a great number of complexly learned inhibitions of drive aims. Psychoanalysis posits, for instance, that the earliest and most severe learned inhibitive behavior (often appearing self-punitive) stems from the anal phase, related to excessive cleanliness training. That is, a child severely trained to be clean may be excessively afraid of any "dirtiness" (including verbal abuse), may grow up into an adult always feeling "dirty" (guilty), and may suffer from an "inner voice of conscience" which is the persistent unconscious apperception of the nagging and reprimanding voice or look of the mother. In this sense "moral masochism" may be understood as a continuous effect of apperception of such an "anal-sadistic" mother upon one's apperception of one's contemporary feeling, thinking, and behavior.

I hasten to emphasize that psychoanalytic hypotheses are by no means so naive or oversimplified as to assume that cleanliness training is in a one-to-one relationship to the formation of the superego, or for that matter that it constitutes all of the causal factors. On the contrary, there are dozens of factors. The learning involved in the correct apperceptions of the dangers of the oedipus constellation, and the related inhibition of aims directed toward mother as object become a powerful further contribution to the set of regulators.

The apperceptions pertaining to the superego appear in pure culture—in the hallucinations of a schizophrenic whose voices may accuse him, frequently in a clearly parental voice, of any number of infractions. Similarly, the self-accusations of the melancholic can be understood in linear continuity (instead of appearing senseless) if one interpolates the sets of hypotheses psychoanalysis has postulated for this syndrome, with particular reference to a distortion of the patient's contemporary feelings or behavior by past apperceptions associated with control and punishment for aggressive aims.

Psychoanalytic Theory: "Types" and "Traits"

Thus far, I have stated that (1) psychoanalytic theory provides a richer than usual trait theory because, as can be seen in libido theory, a focus on the body and on development is added; and (2) a trait conceptualization brings into relief the importance of libidinal aims. I now add that, considered by the standards of what one might reasonably want from a trait theory, psychoanalysis permits infinitely richer understanding and predictions of many personality characteristics than, for instance, the various inventory approaches described in the first part of the chapter. This can be seen by discussing how psychoanalysis depicts personality types. In accordance with my view of science, I will attempt to express some of these psychoanalytic views as propositions, laying out the logical structure of the depictions.

The main dynamic syndromes that one may identify as constituting psychoanalytically formulated personality types are the oral personality, the anal personality, the phallic type, and the urethral type. This classification is primarily founded on the genetic dynamic propositions of the libido theory. However, predicated on the outstanding pathological trait, personality types are often also referred to by analysts as the "phobic" or the "obsessive-compulsive" type of personality, or the "voyeuristic," or the "exhibitionistic." Similarly, *oral, anal,* and *phallic* are used as adjectives to refer to personality traits, and, incidentally, need not imply a clinical disorder. These traits may be integrated aspects of the character structure that lead neither to subjective discomfort nor to objective impairment, but simply constitute modes of operations that discernably have more of an organizing effect on an individual's behavior than other characteristics he possesses.

Psychoanalysis has advanced the concept of "anal character," for example, to describe a personality in which anal traits are outstanding in a nonpathological way.* Such character *types* are not always clearly differentiated, but should be, from character *disorder,* in which the same traits exist to an extent that they cause difficulties to the environment (e.g., to the patient's wife, or husband, or employer) and get the patient into difficulty with the environment without inherently causing him subjective discomfort. The psychoneurosis (e.g., a compulsive neurosis), on the other hand, is characterized primarily by subjective difficulties—primarily in that clinically admixtures of character disorder and psychoneurosis are very frequent.

The concept of "oral personality," for example, permits one the following basic propositions (we are not differentiating further into active and passive oral):

1. *Behavioral propositions*: An excessive response to food (overeating, usually with anorexia under specific circumstances); impulsiveness; passive-dependent behavior with a great need for affection; low frustration tolerance; little patience; mood swings; flexibility, often including inventiveness, hand in hand with carelessness.

2. *Pathological propositions*: Tendency toward depression; use of mechanism of denial and elation; obesity; frequently premature ejaculation in males; great sensitivity of feelings, the tendency to be easily hurt.

3. *Genetic propositions (postdictums)*: A childhood deprived of affection in any number of ways. This may be difficult to quantify except by rank ordering a number of people. It should then be possible on the basis of such rank

---

*As a test of the anal trait hypothesis, I suggest taking a sample of bankers or accountants and matching them with a group of firefighters. I predict that the incidence of bedwetting and/or premature ejaculation will be much higher among the firefighters and the incidence of constipation much higher among the bankers/accountants.

ordering of deprivation (all other things being equal) to predict degree of oral characteristics, which could easily be experimentally investigated (frustration tolerance, etc.).

Actually, the above example is but a short schematic presentation; much more complex propositions can be derived simply from the diagnosis, "severe oral type": The wish to devour, the wish to be devoured, and the wish to sleep constitute a syndrome. Thus, oral people usually like to sleep, in adversity may take to sleeping long and frequently, and if depressed may wish to be dead. This idea of death is almost always equated with sleeping peacefully. Diagnostically, this can be of the greatest importance, since this type of suicidal idea in the absence of other characteristics is usually benign in distinction to other such ideas.

Similar to the oral type or trait, the other traits involve complex propositions that interlock with other concepts concerning defenses, relations to objects, and every other variable of personality. Research establishing the trait clustering as postulated by psychoanalysis will not be enough. Prediction of complex experimental behavior should go further to verify and enlarge the usefulness of these concepts.

The Future

Scientific progress is affected by far too many factors to predict with any certainty. Yet, if the genetic inheritance of traits can shake off its association with unsavory racial theories, then progress in genetics and microbiology will shed light on constitutional contributions to character. We now know that temperament is one of the most stable features of a person's lifelong development. Data have been collected that point to remarkable resemblances in the personalities of identical twins reared apart. I only hope that if this progress comes, and, as is usually the case, new conceptualizations are needed, those involved will look to the resources available through psychoanalysis.

CHAPTER FIVE

Psychoanalysis as Developmental Theory

Introduction

The core of the classic psychoanalytic theory of development was the libido theory. Prior to Freud, *libido* in medical science referred to a person's sexual interests in a specific context. If, for instance, a patient was suffering from an endocrine disorder associated with gross pathological effects on his sexual life, he would be referred to as suffering from increased or deficient libido. This usage of the term continues today.

Freud, however, gave *libido* a technical meaning as well—namely, drive energy. After Freud, Karl Abraham influenced the development of the term. A well-trained embryologist before he became a psychiatrist and psychoanalyst, Abraham applied some concepts of segmental development to his new field and conceived of an orderly sequence of stages of libidinal development, from the oral zone (active and passive) to the anal zone (retentive and aggressive-ejective) to the genital. Thus the libido theory is to a certain extent concerned with maturational processes. In addition, the theory includes the effect of upbringing and relative emphasis or frustration of the various zones and aims; the timing of the stimulation (earlier or later in life); the subsequent effects on the personality in terms of fixation, regression, symptom formation, and object relationships; and the reversibility of any adverse effects.

As I see the matter, there is nothing mysterious about the notions involved. Recalling the logical positivist emphasis on orderly structure, I can state the libido theory as a series of interlocking propositions:

1. Propositions concerning the sequence of maturation of bodily zones with a positive hedonic tone (erotogenic zones) and specific aims of gratification (libidinal aims)
2. Propositions concerning the perception of oral, anal, and genital stimuli and the reaction of significant figures to such stimlulation (early anal training, masturbation, and prohibition)
3. Propositions concerning specific effects on later development of the maturation of learned aspects (object relations, character formation)
4. Propositions concerning the timing of maturation and learning (e.g., the same maternal act at different times in a child's life will have different effects)
5. Propositions concerning the interaction of events learned at different times (the relationship of trauma sustained in infancy to trauma sustained in latency to trauma sustained in puberty)

All these propositions are conceived quantitatively—in terms of a constitutional variation of the strength of drives, variations in the strength of stimluation or lack of stimulation, and quantitative differences in the nature of learning.

Of course, libido theory has now become one model among many. Although I still retain a tie to it, my primary allegiance is, as always, to the linkage between empirical work and model making. In the next section, I address the current status of this linkage.

Current Status

Nearly every psychoanalyst would agree with me that development is important, but there is very little agreement about how to study it. As with so many other subjects, some analysts believe it must be studied on the couch, by using the patient's associations to reconstruct his psychological past, tracing relations between developmental events and later psychological structures. From a scientific point of view, this approach leaves something to be desired; the data are both extremely complicated and subject to many influences at once. Also, even the most neutral analyst will often influence the path taken by a patient's thoughts and, consequently, the developmental story that emerges.

There is a certain irony to the current situation. Most people who follow developmental literature would agree that we have learned an enormous amount about the early period of human life. We have a better understanding of how affect comes to be regulated, how social relations develop, and how cognition and language build on early skills. Yet, despite this solid body of knowledge, analysts are locked in heated disagreements with one another about how to use it. I suspect that all this heat is generated because some fear that the new knowledge will force them to choose between their cherished "developmental" theories, based on their clinical work, and scientific findings from infant observation. Perhaps some analysts are afraid of an identity crisis—they worry that if they give up some traditional psychoanalytic ideas, they can no longer consider themselves to be psychoanalysts.

In Freud's time, when the scientific study of development was in its infancy, this conflict seems not to have bothered anyone.

Freud's Early Sightings of Development

I suppose the earliest psychoanalytic pronouncement on development was the now famous observation that "hysterics suffer mainly from reminiscences" (Breuer & Freud, 1895). As usual, Freud liked to claim that his interest in the patient's past was something forced on him by the evidence (in this case, the clinical evidence that "demanded" he reconstruct earlier feeling states and experiences). But it seems reasonable to believe that Freud brought with him a real tendency to sift through the data, looking for evidence of the effects of the past.

Why might Freud have been inclined to look to childhood for answers about psychopathology? First, in Freud's medical training, as in mine, one was taught to begin with a careful anamnesis (case history). Second, Freud's youthful political convictions continued into his early psychoanalytic days, expressing themselves in the hope that psychoanalysis might contribute to needed social reforms, especially in education and child rearing. So, developmental theory was needed to provide a basis for sounder practices. Third, and probably most important, was a rather unspecific cultural and personal attitude. Sociologist Philip Reiff said that whereas for Marx the present was pregnant with the future, for Freud the present was pregnant with the past. If you have seen a photograph of Freud's consulting room, then you have seen his desk piled high with archeological antiquities and the like—testimony to a cultural conviction that the past is the source of the present. I imagine Freud would have agreed with the southern writer, William Faulkner, who used his novels to show how the past continues to exert its influence in the present. (Responding to the suggestion that the past is dead, a Faulkner character says that not only is the past not dead, it isn't even the past yet.)

Even if Freud felt certain that an individual's past was important, he did not usually take much interest in the direct study of development. However, there are two exceptions worth noting. W. Ernst Halberstadt-Freud (my boyhood friend) was the most famous baby in the history of psychoanalytic infant observation. The son of Freud's daughter, Sophie, Ernst appeared in *Beyond the Pleasure Priniciple* (1920), where Freud described Ernst's attempt to master by active mimicry the painful rhythm of his mother's comings and goings. You recall how he first tossed from his crib, then retrieved, a wooden object attached to a string. As he amused himself with this gravely serious drama, he labeled what happened, saying "o-o-o-o" for *fort* ("gone") when he threw out the spool and *da* ("there") when he brought it back to him (Freud, 1920, pp. 14–15).

(As an aside, it is interesting to note how Freud's little anecdote about Ernst resembles later research. It is naturalistic, not experimental. That is, it watches a child being childlike in a familiar setting without trying too hard to control variables responsible for an action. And, as was to prove so important in subsequent research, this study of a child was really a study of a child-in-relation-to-a-mother and, more particularly, a study of a child negotiating a separation. These themes—the effort to collect data from real-life situations and to pay attention to the child's relation to a caregiver—are hallmarks of much later research.)

A second exception to Freud's general tendency to move from adult clinical evidence to reconstructed development was his secondhand child analysis of Herbert Graf, known to posterity as "Little Hans" in Freud's *Analysis of a Phobia in a Five-Year-Old Boy* (1909).

Herbert's father, the well-known musicologist Max Graf, was an early member of Freud's Wednesday Psychological Society (though he later withdrew) and his mother was an early patient of Freud's. As convinced Freudians, they tried to raise Herbert in a way consistent with psychoanalysis. The result of their earnest efforts was sometimes amusing, as when his mother evidently felt compelled to reinforce, with a verbal threat, Herbert's castration anxiety. She once scolded him, warning him that the doctor would come and cut off his penis. (Herbert's mother could have saved both of them the trouble. This anxiety usually needs no such coaxing. Freud had predicted this fear happens naturally—and pretty much inevitably—for essentially developmental reasons.)

Freud visited Herbert on his third birthday and met him for a consultation in the course of an "analysis" conducted by the elder Graf when the boy developed a fear that a horse would bite him. The method adopted called for the father to interview the boy, then report to Freud. Freud offered interpretations, which in turn influenced the father's interactions and statements to the boy. The details of the analysis (which I recommend to the reader) are best understood in the case itself, but evidence for the successful resolution, by this unusual "analysis," of the (mostly oedipal) conflicts at work can be found in an equally unusual opportunity to see the outcome of the case. In 1922, a nineteen- year-old Herbert Graf visited Freud. He had shown emotional resilience in coming through his parents' divorce without obvious psychological injury, and he later became well known in his own right, following in his father's footsteps by becoming a producer and director of operas in New York, Philadelphia, and Zurich (Gay, 1988, pp. 255–260; Clark, 1980, p. 236).

Freud on Developmental Theory

Although these bits of data from Ernst and from Herbert Graf certainly broaden the usual picture of Freud's thinking on development—and make it possible for contemporary developmental researchers to claim a connection to Freud—it would be a mistake to make too much of them. In general, what Freud had to say about development was a reconstruction based on clinical evidence. When he elaborated it in his theory, he tended to derive his developmental stages and generalizations from psychoanalytic principles, not from direct observation of children, and certainly not from controlled experimental examination of their responses.

We get a more accurate picture of Freud's use of observational data if we acknowledge that these two observational data sets probably would not have found a place in his writings had they not fit so neatly with ideas he had already developed.

When Freud told the story of Ernst's *fort-da* game, he

freely admitted he took advantage of what he called the "chance opportunity" to observe Ernst and that "no certain decision can be reached on the analysis of a single case" (1920, pp. 14, 16). In the context of the entire book, it is clear that Freud had a strong rhetorical motive for recounting his observation. He hoped the reader would feel puzzled enough by Ernst's repetition of a painful experience to listen to Freud's case for influences other than (and beyond) the pleasure principle. I find it hard to believe that Freud would have told the story if Ernst's behavior was more in line with the theory he was abandoning, rather than the one he was formulating. I doubt he would have noticed it at all.

In 1919, Freud wrote to Ernest Jones about the "Little Hans" case that "I never got a finer insight into a child's soul." His enthusiasm for child observation should be understood in the context of its ability to illustrate the stages and principles in his *Three Essays on a Theory of Sexuality* (Freud, 1905), which he had just finished (letter cited in Gay, 1988, pp. 255–256).

In *Three Essays,* one gets the classic psychoanalytic view of developmental stages, expressed in scientific form, but without an eye toward specific falsifiable predictions. Freud devoted one essay apiece to three topics: "The Sexual Abberrations," "Infantile Sexuality," and "Transformations of Puberty." They are interesting to read because, here and there, one can catch a glimpse of the reformist zeal I mentioned earlier. By this time, the zeal showed itself as Freud's plain-spoken willingness to shock the sexually unenlightened sensibilities of his bourgeois readership. Doubly offensive is the point that the so-called perversions are extreme expressions of psychological elements found in earlier stages of even the most conventional upbringing. With this pronouncement, Freud not only connected perversion with normality, he also located it in the stage of life most often thought to be innocent. Thus the hypothesis of a developmental history, in which the earlier mental stages that have been superseded are organized around now repressed thoughts and feelings, accomplished two important purposes: It argued for the continuity of illness and health and it debunked childhood innocence.

The well-known oral, anal, and phallic stages themselves are discussed in more detail in Chapter Four, but a brief summary may be appropriate. In the first section of that chapter, I described the view of libido as a mobile instinctual energy, capable of being attached (cathected) to various psychologically important objects. In determining the course of these attachments, Freud brought together clinical observations of the correlations of traits, pathologies, speculations regarding child rearing, and physiological evidence regarding the distribution of nerve tissue in the body. The first erogenous zone is the mouth. The child takes pleasure in eating, sucking his thumb, and putting objects in the mouth. The next zone is the anus. The child takes pleasure in bowel activity, both holding in and expelling his feces, along with the control this gives him over his caregivers. The third is the phallus (or clitoris). The child takes pleasure in masturbation. Longings for the same and opposite sexed parent develop into an oedipal conflict.

In the boy, the transfer of libido to the phallus gives a specific intensity to his already heated attachment to his mother. Fantasies take on a more explicitly sexual form, including what he understands to constitute intercourse. At the same time, a countervailing force is the castration anxiety so vividly embodied by Frau Graf's threat to Herbert that the doctor would cut off his penis. Freud also speculated that, on seeing female genitalia, the oedipal child concludes that they are the result of castration; the combination of threats, fantasies, and childish theories leads the oedipal youngster to see castration as a serious danger. This fear is combined with the perception that the chief rival for the mother's affection is, of course, the powerful and ominous father. Usually the fear overwhelms the rivalry and the boy comes to identify with the father. Thus the child introduces into his mind an internal prohibition against access to the mother, and so he is protected from acting on a impulse that he senses would lead him to a disaster in the real world.

The Next Generation: Anna Freud and Melanie Klein

My psychoanalytic training was interrupted by the Anschluss, but had I been able to continue, my first case would have been one of a child analysis supervised by Aichkorn. The reason for this was my young age. It was generally accepted that a young analyst would have difficulty commanding the respect needed for the analysis of an older (and possibly socially superior) adult. Women analysts were steered toward child analysis for much the same reason.

From our perspective today, we can see this as a prejudice, perhaps even a form of discrimination. It may be all the more amusing to look at the result of this mentality, which thought of women, young analysts, and child analysts as somehow second class. Because Freud's daughter, Anna, was a child analyst, the practice of child analysis enjoyed a period of protection. It was established that the data gained from children were at least as valuable a source of information about development as were the reconstructions from the associations of an adult patient.

Child analysis paved the way for the direct study of child development by psychoanalysts. Although child analysis was clinically focused, the reconstructions of development did not have to reach far back into the past. And the fact that disturbed youngsters will not sit still made it inevitable that child analysts watch behavior as well as listen to associations. (In child analysis, children are usually allowed to draw, play with toys, and so on while the analyst watches, asks questions, and offers interpretations.) Also, from the start, child analysis combined prophylactic and curative goals. This factor also shifted the data somewhat, for it meant that the developmental observations had a less decided bias toward the pathological than did Freud's reconstructions from adult data. I mention these two shifts—the movement toward increased observation and the diminished focus on pathological forms—because, as we shall see in later sections, they were to prove the wave of the future.

Anna Freud

Neither a physician nor a professional academic, Anna Freud was a gifted clinician and educator who, quite early in her career, gravitated to the two dominating interests of her life: caring for children and for her father (and his legacy). She was involved with Siegfried Bernfeld's Kinderheim Baumgarten, a Jewish camp for homeless children and, later, with two child guidance centers (Grosskurth, 1986). In defiance of every guideline of psychoanalysis, she was analyzed by her father. She became a member of the Vienna Society in June of 1922, reading as her membership paper, "The Relationship of Beating-Phantasies to a Day-Dream," using, Young-Breuhl has argued, disguised material from her own childhood and adolesence. And, not surprisingly, she drew increasingly closer to her father as he proved unable to find a surrogate son among his followers. In 1927, she published *Einführung in die Technik der Kinderanalyse*.

Anna Freud was soon embroiled in controversy, largely as a result of disagreements with the followers of Melanie Klein, whose ideas I will describe below. As Anna Freud saw the matter, a fundamental aspect of the dispute involved what to make of some of the differences between child and adult analysis. Unlike the adult who (more or less) chooses analysis, the child is placed into it by parents seeking relief. The analyst is therefore obliged to win the child's confidence, even to the point of fostering positive dependency. Working with children, the analyst must relax many of the conventional standards. For example, some child analysts offer snacks or a drink at the end of a session as a reward for the work done and as a way of building positive associations.

Technical recommendations like these obviously depend on implicit developmental theories. For example, theoretical differences with Klein dictated different interpretations of the child's hostility or tenderness toward the analyst. Anna Freud thought that a child who is tenderly attached to the mother will be wary of outsiders, including the analyst. Thus the wariness is not a transference copy of the child's feeling toward the parent so much as it is a consequence of a quite different feeling. Klein, on the other hand, tended to interpret the child's feelings toward the analyst as a reflection of his feelings toward the parent.

Melanie Klein

Melanie Klein, a nonmedical analyst who emigrated to Great Britain, promoted a different (and antagonistic) view of child analysis. She rejected an educational approach for a more aggressively analytic one. Like Anna Freud, Klein was the daughter of a physician. She had intended to study medicine but stopped her studies when she married at an early age. (She was, however, divorced soon afterwards.) Living in Budapest between 1910 and 1919, she was attracted to Freud by his writings and sought out psychoanalytic treatment from the well-known Hungarian analyst Sandor Ferenczi. Ferenczi suggested she apply analytic techniques to children. She attracted interest when reports of her work reached the wider psychoanalytic community. She was invited to Berlin by Karl Abraham, where a brief analysis followed. In 1925, Ernest Jones invited her to present her findings in Great Britain and she soon settled there.

Sponsorship by three such prominent analysts undoubtedly gave a boost to her work, comparable in kind, if not in extent, to the boost given Anna Freud by her association with her father. Considered together, the interest shown in both early branches of child analysis ensured its findings would be read with interest and attention.

The terms of the split between Anna Freud and Melanie Klein were not initially clear, especially since Klein insisted that her work was an extension of the older Freud. Undoubtedly, there was a political element in her insistence, but it is quite true that her early work resembled Freud's thoughts about his treatment of Herbert Graf: Both emphasized libidinal issues. In contrast to the prevailing

Freudian view, however, Klein claimed to have found evidence of a much earlier dating of oedipal interests (and, importantly, earlier accompanying superego figures).

Several points should be made about the evidential basis of Klein's findings. Contrary to what is generally assumed, according to a chapter in Greenberg and Mitchell (1983), Klein's conclusions were not the result of observation of pre-oedipal children. Her youngest patient was 31 months old, and most were a good bit older, falling clearly within what is usually defined as the oedipal phase. This fact about her sample is important because although her findings are in one sense the result of observation, they are as much reconstructions as were Freud's reconstructions from adult clinical data. Klein's data are mostly derived from the fantasies of older children.

John Bowlby

Near the close of the same decade that saw Freud publishing his observations of his grandson Ernst, the German edition of Anna Freud's *The Psychoanalytical Treatment of Children* (1926), and the emigration of Melanie Klein to London, a British medical student interested in developmental psychology took a year to work at a school for maladjusted children. There, his curiosity was sparked by an 8-year-old boy who attached himself to the student, following him wherever he went. Bowlby does not say what became of the boy, but the path taken by Bowlby's career shows that his curiosity continued.

Bowlby went from his medical studies at Cambridge to the Institute of Psychoanalysis in London and the London Child Guidance Clinic and Training Center. Analyzed by Joan Riviere and supervised by Melanie Klein, he soon fell into disagreements with them. Once he qualified analytically in 1937, he gave as his membership paper an essay that stressed the influence on the inner life from the real events (rather than fantasies) of childhood: "The Influence of Early Environment on the Development of

Neurosis and Neurotic Character." After his war service, he ran the children's department of Tavistock Institute in London, where he was soon joined by Jimmy Robertson, a psychiatric social worker who collaborated with Bowlby in his most significant research on attachment and separation.

Bowlby and Robertson took a clever first step. As happens so often in a new research area, they felt they first needed to demonstrate that a phenomenon existed that called for an explanation. To do so, Robertson collected data on children between 12 and 36 months old who for one reason or another had been in a hospital or residential nursery. He observed, for example, how many hours they cried, both when they arrived at the new setting and afterwards. Although this method obviously lacked needed controls, it confirmed the beliefs of Bowlby and Robertson and provided them with a brainstorm—a way of communicating their message.

They needed data that were comparatively direct and conducive to dramatic presentation. Bowlby had been impressed by Rene Spitz's 1947 film, *Grief: A Peril in Infancy*, and so Bowlby and Robertson decided a hospital visit should be recorded on film. They produced a documentary of an eight-day hospital stay by a healthy little girl who needed minor corrective surgery on an umbilical hernia. The result was *A Two-Year-Old Goes to Hospital*. It was shown at the Institute of Psychoanalysis on March 5, 1952, and soon became a staple of medical education in Great Britain. (Of course, this film was not subjected to the sort of frame-by-frame analysis that is now common, nor were recording conditions well controlled. The point was to demonstrate that spotting extreme infant distress required little or no inference—however it might be diagnosed.)

In 1950, the World Health Organization asked Bowlby to prepare a report on the mental health of homeless children. He stressed that "What is believed essential for mental health is that the infant and young child should experience a warm, intimate and continuous relationship with his mother (or permanent mother substitute) in which both find satisfaction and enjoyment" (1951, cited in Bowlby, 1969, pp. xi–xii). Both Bowlby and reviewers of the report felt unsatisfied because, however clear it might be that maternal deprivation was harmful, little or no scientific evidence existed to throw light on the processes at work.

In pursuing this matter, Bowlby was assisted by contact with new theories and further empirical studies. In the summer of 1951, a psychologist at the London School of Economics urged Bowlby to take a look at Konrad Lorenz's studies of the tendency of baby geese to follow their mother. He started with a translation of a 1935 German paper. Bowlby knew the famous biologist Julian Huxley and asked him about Lorenz; upon Huxley's enthusiastic endorsement, Bowlby threw himself into the emerging literature on ethology, the study of animal behavior.

In June 1957, he presented a paper that used ethological ideas to explain his human subject matter: "The Nature of the Child's Tie to His Mother" (Grosskurth, 1986, p. 403). Instead of accepting Anna Freud's idea of a secondary drive (a "cupboard love") responsible for the attachment, or Klein's emphasis on oral factors, Bowlby postulated a primary tendency to stay close to a special figure, much as one sees in infant monkeys. Furthermore, if this tendency is an innate potential elicited by life experiences, then one is able to explain diverse behaviors, such as crying, clinging, smiling, and the like, as modes by which the attachment is realized. (As I shall describe below, Bowlby met mostly with angry rejection.)

Between 1958 and 1963, he elaborated and extended his application of ethology in several papers: "Separation Anxiety," "Grief and Mourning in Infancy," "Processes of Mourning," "Pathological Mourning," and "Childhood Mourning." (Unless the reader has a genuinely historical interest, it is probably best to read about these ideas in Bowlby's three volumes of *Attachment and Loss.*)

At Tavistock, further studies were conducted that introduced better experimental controls. Christoph Heinicke (1956) and Heinicke and Ilse Westheimer (1966) repeated the earlier observations of children separated from family, this time using matched samples for comparisons and statistical analysis of the resuling data.

Many variations have been found in the basic pattern detected, but it was found overall that a child of 15 to 30 months with a fairly secure attachment to his mother shows a predictable sequence of three phases: protest, despair, and detachment. During the protest phase, which may either begin immediately or be delayed, the young child is acutely distressed, crying loudly, shaking, throwing his body back and forth, and eagerly looking toward any sound. The observer sees the suggestion that the child strongly expects the mother to return and exercises his full faculties to cause this return. Such a child is likely to reject alternative figures, though some will cling to a nurse.

During the despair phase, which may come into play from within hours to a week or even more, the child continues to be preoccupied with the absence of the mother, yet the decreasing activity level suggests an increasing hopelessness. He cries monotonously and is withdrawn, quiet, and much less demanding.

During the detachment phase, which comes next, the child begins to show more interest in the environment. He accepts nursing care, food, and toys. To some extent, increased sociability is present. Superficially considered, the behavioral evidence seems to indicate a return to a previous level of sociability and activation—with one critically important and striking exception. When the mother visits, the child fails to react with the strong attachment behavior normal at his age. He fails to greet the mother, does not cling, and seems remote, apathetic, and listless. Less striking, but just as ominous for future development, is a trend noticeable over time with children who have gone through repetitions of the loss through transient attachments to nurses. The child comes to care less about human contact and more about material things (candies, toys, etc.). The resulting sociability may seem cheerful but it is notably shallow, without real caring.

Two kinds of arguments resulted from these findings. One kind of argument accepted the general framework and legitimacy of the research program, but disputed the weight attached to various causal variables and definition of the phases. It was suggested that the children were upset by the strange environment or that the previous relationship with the mother was defective; it was not the separation *per se* that caused the reactions. This issue has been debated and attempts have been made to tease out necessary and sufficient conditions for the response. Bowlby continues to believe that the most weighty factor is the separation itself.

Another kind of argument was launched by Bowlby's opponents within British psychoanalysis, who challenged the appropriateness of the framework he brought to his studies. The reader needs first to know that the British Psychoanalytic Society has been historically quite factionalized, divided among those loyal to Anna Freud's ideas (the "A" group), those loyal to Melanie Klein's ideas (the "B" group), and a third group of those who choose neither side (the "middle" group). (Needless to say, I find such factionalization contrary to the scientific spirit but it does make interesting reading. The reader can find it described in the biographies of Melanie Klein by Phyllis Grosskurth [1986] and of Anna Freud by Elizabeth Young-Breuhl [1988].)

Just prior to the meeting in which Bowlby presented his first use of ethological evidence, he gave a copy of his address to a colleague he considered a friend. When he presented the paper, he found himself not only criticized, which he had expected, but he also found the Kleinian group lying in wait for him, evidently with prior knowledge of his arguments. Anna Freud did not attend, but based on what she learned of his paper, she wrote to Donald Winnicott (another prominent British analyst), worrying that "Dr. Bowlby is too valuable a person to get lost to psychoanalysis" (Grosskurth, 1986, p. 404).

There were, of course, many reasons given for the unacceptability of Bowlby's approach to development, but they usually boiled down to this belief: He had parted company with psychoanalysis because he used biobehavioral data without bringing it into a metapsychological framework (i.e., translating it into the language of id, ego, superego, and various unconscious processes). However, the emotional component behind many of the complaints may have been better expressed in the lament of British analyst Dr. A. Hyatt Williams, who stated that Bowlby "took the poetry out of analysis" (Grosskurth, 1986, p. 406).

I would agree with Bowlby that this is no criticism. When it comes to analysis, we would do best to let science have the last word whenever possible. When advancing our knowledge of development, we must not stop to worry about the level of poetry we leave behind.

Margaret Mahler

Margaret Mahler began her medical career in Vienna as a pediatrician and came to the United States in the late 1930s. Mahler's views underwent various revisions and changes in the use of terms and dates for phases, but a practical systematic formulation can be found in *The Psychological Birth of the Human Infant* (Mahler, Pine, & Bergman, 1975). My summary draws on that book and on the description given in *Object Relations in Psychoanalytic Theory* (Greenberg & Mitchell, 1983).

Mahler's research started out with a tendency to concentrate on what developmental studies can teach us about psychopathology. In her first studies, she searched for the developmental sources of certain psychotic states. She had written on this topic as early as the late 1940s, but her major research came in a series of projects in the 1950s and 1960s, funded mostly by the National Institute for Mental Health, which sought to extend her ideas from the examination of developmental precursors of psychopathology to normal development.

The data reported in *Psychological Birth* were collected in a pilot (1959–1962) and a more formal study (1962–1968) of 38 children and their 22 mothers, along with subsequent intensive investigation of some of the children in the latter group. Mother-child pairs were observed in specially designed rooms.

A number of methods were used to increase the power of the observations to function as data. Participant observers were encouraged to rely on their empathic, clinical sense of what was happening, although they were also asked to note evidence for any inferences. Notes were recorded for each session. Nonparticipant observers watched from behind a one-way mirror for a period of about a half hour. Later in the study, the nonparticipant observer was asked to coordinate his account with the participant observer, so that two perspectives were available on the same sample of behavior.

Ratings were tried but not found to be feasible. Instead, "area observations" were used. Observers commented on such specific areas as locomotor activity, vocalization, affect, and so on. The nonparticipant observer was kept separate from the other staff for a year, in order to avoid contamination of observations.

Mothers were interviewed weekly, fathers less systematically. Film records and home visits were made. Both children and their mothers were psychologically tested. Two kinds of staff conferences were held: a semiweekly staff conference attended by all staff other than the isolated nonparticipant observer and research conferences by the senior investigators.

Quite a bit of data were collected. Along the way, hypotheses were developed, modified, or discarded. Data-collection methods were revised, sometimes in response to new ideas, sometimes because more mundane considerations of money or time required cutbacks. What were the findings?

The infant begins with the normal autistic phase (see Box 5–1). For several weeks, he functions as a closed system, sleeping often, aroused rarely, and relatively removed from the external world. This system is dominated by tension reduction, using hallucinatory wish fulfillment. The infant has not yet sufficiently activated and awakened the sense organs by which he is to be attached to the world.

BOX 5–1 • *Mahler's Developmental Sequence*

Forerunners of the Separation-Individuation Process
Normal Autistic Phase
Normal Symbiotic Phase

Separation-Individuation Subphases

Differentiation and the Development of the Body Image
Practicing
Rapprochement
Individuality Consolidation and Start of Object Constancy

Based on Mahler, Pine, and Bergman, 1975.

Experience is little more than the ebb and flow of homeostatic regulation.

Near the close of the first month, increased sensitivity to external stimulation pushes the infant into the normal symbiotic phase. The mother appears, if only as a source able to aid in tension regulation. Attention turns tentatively outward, toward the periphery, though, for the infant, this periphery marks no break, as he experiences the union with the mother as undivided. Experience, however, is divided; good, pleasurable memory traces are grouped together and bad, unpleasant memory traces are grouped together. Simple anticipations appear of the structure, which will later be organized as self and other.

Starting at about four or five months, separation-individuation begins. It comes in subphases. First is the *differentiation* subphase. Mahler says it begins with "hatching." Wakefulness is fully alert for the first time. Instead of relaxing his body into the form of the caregiver's hold, the infant begins to position himself. Exploration begins. Baby grabs mother's hair, face, and clothes. The infant visually explores the world he will enter, preparing for and then initiating his exit from the caregiver's lap. Discrimination appears, as does stranger anxiety.

Next is the *practicing* subphase, composed of early practicing and practicing subphase proper. Now able to crawl, the child can move away from the caregiver. He does so, but without abandoning use of the caregiver as a base. The child gets a sense of the independence of his own body, develops a new emotional bond to the caregiver, and strengthens his ego capacities.

With these early powers in place, the psychological birth begins in earnest when the child assumes the upright position. He sees more and acts more—and takes pleasure in his new power to see and to act. But, Mahler says, the child does not yet know the mother to be a separate entity.

This exhilaration soon subsides. In the *rapprochement* subphase, during the middle of the second year, it begins to dawn on the child that the increasing autonomy in fact indicates that the caregiver may not always be available. Separation anxiety sets in. Things are very tough; the child is caught in a bind. He needs outside help and is quite vulnerable to frustration. Yet outside help can undermine his developing capacities. The child can be damned if he gets help and damned if he doesn't. It is perhaps for this reason that Mahler sees the surmounting of the crises during this period as the precondition for freedom from severe psychopathology.

During the third year, there comes the phase of libidinal object constancy, during which the child (and later the adult) must organize stable concepts of self and other. This stage is open ended in Mahler's system.

The Contemporary Scene

Despite the diversity of developmental approaches, a few trends can be identified. There has been a steady movement away from sole reliance on after-the-fact reconstruction of childhood, a reconstruction based on adult memories and supplemented by psychoanalytic theory. Analysts and others observed children, hoping to confirm Freudian hypotheses that linked certain adult pathologies to specific stages of development, and also hoping to refine their knowledge of pathogenic mechanisms in childhood.

Two largely unforeseen results followed. Freud said there was a continuum between pathology and normal functioning. It made very little sense to try to identify a given developmental event as pathogenic unless there was some basis of comparison, and so normal development needed to be observed. Also, analysts soon discovered that data collected to confirm or refine analytic hypotheses can just as easily end up challenging those hypotheses. Soon, observational data began to be used to challenge the developmental theories that had been built up mostly from reconstructions. These changes have forced those bent on remaining loyal Freudians to make some tough choices.

Dan Stern

These changes can be understood by examining an ambitious, quite controversial book written recently by an analyst committed to using empirical developmental evidence to make some hard demands on psychoanalytic theory. This book is *The Interpersonal World of the Infant* by Dan Stern (1985). The mission he has set himself is well described by the subtitle of his book: *A View from Psychoanalysis and Developmental Psychology*.

Formerly Chief of the Laboratory of Developmental Processes at Cornell University Medical Center and now at Brown University, Stern is a psychiatrist with an unusually sophisticated knowledge of the techniques of developmental research. He has drawn on this combination of clinical and scientific perspectives in his work.

In the preface of his book, he describes an incident from his childhood. When he was about 7 years old, he watched an adult struggling to deal with an infant of 1 or 2 years. As he watched, he felt he understood what the infant was all about, yet the adult seemed uncomprehending. Stern was part of both worlds, still young enough to know in his gut the world of the infant, but old enough to communicate with the adult whose world he was slowly entering. He was, Stern recalled, still "bilingual," and wondered if the years to come would oblige him to loose his knowledge of the younger child's "language."

It is impossible not to see his book as an effort to recover what he felt was lost to *him* since that time. Again and again, he calls on the most up-to-date observational data, yet his purpose is not simply to craft a theory. He wishes to capture the subjective, live reality of infancy and restore, as much as possible, that 7-year-old's sense of knowing *from the inside* what the infant was about.

In the course of this personal quest, he also seeks out a new—and, I suspect, inherently unstable—joining together of what he calls the "observed infant" of the infant observation laboratory and the "clinical infant" reconstructed by psychoanalysis on the basis of clinical material. Stern freely acknowledges that "the problem raised by drawing upon these two differently derived infants is, to what extent are they really about the same thing?" (1985, p. 14). Despite the problems, he gives three reasons to bring the two together: (1) We assume that observable events are somehow transformed into subjective experiences (without this assumption, how could we ever hope to grasp the genesis of psychopathology?); (2) Therapists who are better acquainted with the observed infant may be better able to assist the patient in clinical reconstructions of developmental histories; and (3) The laboratory observer who is familiar with the clinically reconstructed infancy may be better able to observe.

Stern explicitly associates his work with that of previous developmental theorists, including Melanie Klein, John Bowlby, and Margaret Mahler, giving special attention to their emphasis on the importance of the infant's relations with caregivers. And, like Klein and Mahler, he focuses on the infant's experience of self and other. However, Stern takes issue with two prevailing trends I have described so far: Stern quotes with approval a criticism from an article by Peterfreund (1978). This article attacks "two fundamental conceptual fallacies, especially characteristic of psychoanalytic thought: the adultomorphization of infancy and the tendency to characterize early states of normal development in terms of hypotheses about the later states of psychopathology" (p. 427, cited in Stern, 1985, p. 19).

Stern believes that errors have been created by the tendency of preceding generations of psychoanalysts to function as "developmental theorists working backward in time," trying to understand childhood and adult psychopathological states by connecting each with the occurrence of a correlated entity in infancy (1985). Moreover, Stern charges, a backwards-looking theory that describes development as a succession of phase-specific clinical issues—whether it is called orality, separation, or establishment of trust—is simply not equal to the task of accounting for the infant's dramatic, hit-you-over-the-head qualitative leaps in interpersonal relatedness that are universally observed by scientist and parent alike.

Stern illustrates a widespread problem with existing theories by pointing to some of the measurement issues that have figured prominently in this book. As a scientist, he knows that if he wants to locate in time the emotionally crucial development of the infant's sense of independence and autonomy from the caregiver, the answer he gets will depend to a very large extent on what he designates as the observable sign of such independence. Freud (1905) and Erikson (1950) looked to the establishment of independent bowel control, at around age 24 months. Spitz (1957) emphasized a verbal sign familiar to every mother, the child's ability to say "no," coming into place at around 15 months. As discussed earlier, Mahler, Pine, and Bergman (1975) stressed the new vistas open to the child once he can stand erect and wander at will, commencing at around 12 months.

Here, we see variation in dating that amounts to a year, which, in the life of a 2-year-old, is quite a bit of variability. As Stern sees it, however, these differences are not really competing hypotheses that need to be formulated and submitted to a critical test; rather, each is *right in its own way.*

Moreover, there are other equally plausible signs that can be measured and used to date independence. Videotaping has made it possible to document and analyze the ways infant and caregiver gaze at one another, finding striking anticipations of the patterns later found in locomotor behavior. Between 3 and 6 months of age, when the poorly coordinated infant is unable to walk and has only rudimentary hand-eye coordination, his visual system is virtually mature. The infant may not be able to run to his mother or pull away when he is angry, but he can gaze into mother's eyes or refuse her glance.

Even these small babies are able to initiate, maintain, terminate, and avoid engagement with the caregiver through control of their visual systems. One can see them shut down communication by shifting their eyes away, closing them, staring past their partner into space, or becoming glassy-eyed; or invite reengagement by gazing, smiling, or vocalizing. They can take charge of a social situation and regulate the amount of social stimulation they wish to take in at a given moment. When it comes to establishing independence, the infant seems to be engaged in the same back-and-forth of togetherness and separation he will enact 9 months later when he waddles away from and then returns to the side of the caregiver.

What grounds are there in this case for picking the latter period over the former? Sterns asks: Why choose? A more reasonable approach is to go along with something mothers have long known: "Infants can assert their independence and say a decisive 'NO' with gaze aversions at four months, gestures and vocal intonation at seven months, running away at fourteen months, and language at two years" (1985, p. 22). Therefore, Stern finds it more sensible to see clinical issues as lifetime concerns rather than as tied to specific phases.

He does not reject phases altogether, however. Like the academic psychologist, Stern accepts that phases may be designated on the basis of adaptive tasks that arise because of physical and mental maturation. He mentions two important ones, by Sander (1964) and by Greenspan

(1981) (see Box 5–2). The problem with these descriptive systems is that they fail to capture enough of the inner "language" that so fascinated the 7-year-old Stern.

Stern's system concerns the four developing senses of the self: sense of the emergent self, the core self, the subjective self, and the verbal self. First comes the sense of the emergent self, in the first two months of life. This sense of self is an organization beginning to coalesce, not a genuine superordinate self. But this organization is important because it convincingly demonstrates that the assumption of disorganization is simply incorrect.

The scientific revolution that made this finding of organization possible owes as much to technical ingenuity and gadgetry as to theoretical vision. The obstacle to be

---

BOX 5–2 • *Developmental Phases*

Sander (1964)

Physiological regulation	0–3 months
Regulation of reciprocal exchange	3–6 months
Joint regulation of infant initiation in social exchanges and in manipulating the environment	6–9 months
Focalization of activities	10–14 months
Self-assertion	15–24 months

Greenspan (1981)

Homeostasis	0–3 months
Attachment	2–7 months
Somatopsychological differentiation	3–10 months
Behavioral organization, initiative, and internalization	9–24 months
Representational capacity, differentiation, and consolidation	9–24 months

Based on Stern, 1985.

overcome was our difficulty in figuring out how to get very young babies to "answer" our experimental "questions." Fortunately, however, even these vulnerable youngsters come equipped with behaviors in which they excel: head turning, sucking, and looking. MacFarlane (1975), for example, found a way to ask 3-day-olds if they can reliably discriminate the odor of their own mother's milk. He put the infant on his back, with the mother's breast pad on one side and another nursing mother's breast pad on the other side. By varying the way the situation was organized, he discovered that the infant will reliably turn his head to the mother's breast pad, regardless of where it is. Similarly, since infants suck well, psychologists can rig a nipple with a harmless pressure transducer. When the baby sucks at a certain rate, some electrically controlled event will follow (a recorder will go on, a slide carousel will insert a new slide, etc.). This neat trick lets the infant control an event and, in effect, "speak up" for a preference. In this way, it has been found that even in the first weeks of life, infants show a preference for the human voice over other sounds of the same pitch and volume (Freidlander, 1970). And since they can see reasonably well at the right focal distance, their eye movements can also be tracked to discover other "preferences," such as the one they revealed for human faces over other visual patterns.

After the sense of the emergent self comes the sense of the core self. Generally operating outside of awareness, this sense develops between the second and sixth month of life. It concerns the infant's sense that he is a willful, physically separate whole, with distinct affective experiences and a history of his own. The four basic forms of self-experience of this phase are self-agency, self-coherence, self-affectivity, and self-history.

However much psychoanalytic theorists may disagree, this is the period when the world begins to treat the infant as if he had become an integrated self. Stern underlines his split from those theorists (such as Mahler) who describe this phase as a period of slow emergence from an undifferentiated unity with the mother.

An unusual chance event allowed Stern and his staff to verify how their view would fare in a circumstance in which lack of self-differentiation might plausibly be predicted. A pair of so-called "siamese twins" (*Xiphophagus* conjoint twins) was born connected at the ventral surface between the umbilicus and the bottom of the sternum. Though the nervous system of each functioned independently, and they shared no organs and very little blood, they faced one another night and day. Quite often, observers found one or the other or both sucking the fingers of the other twin. Just prior to the surgical separation scheduled for age 4 months (corrected for their prematurity), Stern and his staff tried some gentle experiments to see if, under this unusual circumstance, the two youngsters had difficulty telling which was which. Their method was to remove a finger from the happily sucking mouth and register whether a strain could be detected in the head or arm. By experimentally varying the conditions, they were able to demonstrate that, with these behavioral indices, the infants were never confused about whose finger was being sucked.

Next dawns the sense of the subjective self. The infant realizes that he has a mind and that other people have minds. With this realization comes a growing awareness that the contents of another's mind may be similar enough to his own that the two of them may share the experience. With sharing, of course, comes a new type of relationship. Psychic intimacy is possible, as is the refusal of intimacy. And with this range of possibilities comes the countless decisions of socialization, when caregiver and child negotiate what, when, where, and how aspects of subjectivity will be shared. Among the many important aspects of this new social relatedness, none is more consequential than the caregiver's attunement with the infant, which Stern sees as a "recasting" of the subjective state (1985, p. 161).

Sometime in the second year of life the verbal self emerges. So complex is this change that it cannot be easily paraphrased. Central to this complexity is Stern's insistence on the two-sidedness of the acquisition of language. On the one hand, it greatly increases the child's capacity to make known and share experience. Yet, on the other hand, it "drives a wedge between two simultaneous forms of interpersonal experience: as it is lived and as it is verbally represented" (1985, p. 162). Relatedness, he feels, is moved toward the more impersonal level made possible by language, and away from the immediacy of the other domains of emergent, core, and intersubjective relatedness.

From my description, the reader can easily see the tremendous strides that have been made by researchers studying infants. And just as clearly it can be seen that the data do not speak for themselves. I suspect the challenge for psychoanalysis in the future will be deciding how best to make use of the wealth of findings that have been produced.

CHAPTER SIX

An Operational Definition of the Ego

Introduction

I have never put much stock in the notion that psychoanalysis is a fancy language version of the commonsense wisdom our grandmothers have always understood. However worldly wise our grandmothers may have been, they did not usually acquire their wisdom scientifically, and many of the most important psychoanalytic ideas would strike them as strange.

Consider the notion of the ego, or, as Freud called it in German, *das Ich*. In ordinary German, this phrase means "the I." It is the word President Kennedy used in his famous speech at the Berlin Wall when he identified with his audience, saying, *Ich bin ein Berliner* (I am a Berliner). One of its meanings in Freud is much like the commonsense conception of "the person" or "the self." But Freud also parted company with the commonsense definition, for he also saw *das Ich* as the part of the mind made up of various functions.

The tension between these two approaches is important, as Freud's critics were quick to notice. Stated broadly, the ordinary concept of the person or the self is often taken to imply something unitary, something that cannot be broken into parts as if it were some kind of machine. Those who opposed psychoanalysis seized on Freud's willingness to do so and accused him of being a kind of auto mechanic of the inner life, which the critics viewed as distasteful.

Freud and Ego Psychology

As often happened, Freud changed his mind about the ego—sometimes rather unsystematically. I have summarized this development elsewhere (Bellak, Hurvich, & Gediman, 1973), so I will only mention a few important points. In his unpublished "Project for a Scientific Psychology" (1895), Freud described the ego in organizational terms, as a coherent system that inhibited primary processes. This emphasis on organization never really returned to any important degree.

As is well known, Freud used two systems for dividing up the mind, the so-called *topographic* and *structural* theories. In the first system, Freud spoke of the unconscious, the preconscious, and the conscious. In the second system, he spoke of the id, the ego, and the superego.

The concept of ego instincts was introduced in 1910. At this stage, Freud saw these largely self-preservative functions as in conflict with sexual claims. Ego instincts included cognitive functions, personal ideals, self-protection, and social restrictions, the sorts of functions that further the individual organism's safety and adaptation. When, in *The Ego and the Id* (1923), Freud offered his structural model of the mind, the hypothesis of ego instincts was replaced by the construct of the ego as a mental structure.

Rapaport (1957) stressed some implications of the concept of structure. For example, once a function has been established, it tends to structuralize. That is, it roots itself deeply, eventually stabilizing and ordering its functioning so that any later changes will encounter a certain resistance and therefore proceed slowly. And, once structuralized, a given function tends to organize itself hierarchically.

This way of thinking—viewing the ego as a set of functions—has been criticized on several grounds. Many believe that the definitions of *function* and *structure* depend on one another in a way that makes them suspect. Others find talk of ego functions old fashioned and teleological, the sort of science that might be practiced by Aristotle, explaining the workings of an acorn in terms of the oak it is seeking to become. And even among those who are sympathetic to the ego functional approach, there are caveats: We should not assume that a structure goes with each function or that all functioning is regulated by a structure.

Unless an investigator proceeds carefully, he might make the kind of mistake Molière lampooned—he had a character "explain" how a sleeping potion worked by saying it was effective because of its "soporific properties." If a scientific explanation is to add to knowledge, it must do more than find new ways of saying the same thing; it must find new things to say. And this process requires attention to how terms are defined. In the next sections, I describe how my colleagues and I constructed detailed accounts of the behavioral and psychic operations required to define each ego function, so that they could be reliably identified by different observers.

Ego Functions: A Brief History and Introduction

In *An Outline of Psychoanalysis* (1940), Freud included the following among the principal characteristics of the ego: self-preservation; becoming aware of, and responding to, external stimuli; controlling voluntary movement; learning to influence the external world to one's own advantage through activity; seeking pleasure and avoiding pain; taking account of circumstances in deciding when to satisfy drives; transmitting unexpected increases in unpleasure by an anxiety signal; avoiding overly strong stimuli; remembering; and seeking to reconcile demands from id, superego, and reality sources. Other formulations were given by Anna Freud (1936), Hartmann (1950), and Arlow and Brenner (1964).

My own interest in ego functions goes back to early

preoccupations with schizophrenics. I was much impressed with the fact that some schizophrenics functioned perfectly (e.g., in the area of economics) but were entirely irrational in other everyday affairs. What's more, different schizophrenics seemed to have different ego functions disturbed. I discussed these early impressions in 1949 and 1955 when I developed some attempts to quantify the ego functions. In one of the preliminary research endeavors, several colleagues and myself (Bellak, Hurvich, & Gediman, 1973) attempted to measure seven ego functions in a study of drug effectiveness.

In this study of psychotropic drugs, scales were used to measure the amount of each ego function and its appropriateness. Still, more detailed descriptions were needed if the raters were to agree in their assessments. We wanted to break down each ego function into important components. We decided to treat each ego function as a dimension running from an adaptive end to a maladaptive end so that, for example, we could use the dimension of "reality testing" to compare the person who hears voices with the person who never hears voices, but constantly makes minor mistakes in perceiving what is said to him. (We realized at the time that this was a complicated matter, because using this dimension can be seen as laying down a definition of psychological health—a task that has weighty conceptual and cultural baggage.)

In a later study, funding was obtained from the National Institute of Mental Health to test the usefulness of ego function assessment in describing 50 schizophrenics, 25 neurotics, and 25 normals. (All three groups were similar in age, education, IQ, and socioeconomic status. This similarity allowed us to make comparisons among the groups.)

Twelve major ego functions were selected in the NIMH study. Even then, my colleagues and I realized that there is some overlap among the functions and that a critic might quibble about this or that way of defining a category. Fortunately, the evidence for the reliability and validity of the system gave us confidence that, despite the inevitable element of choice involved in defining a category, the system as a whole was sound.

Some changes were made along the way. The 12 ego functions eventually selected were:

1. *Reality Testing*: The components are (a) the distinction between inner and outer stimuli; (b) the accuracy of perception (including orientation to time and place and interpretation of external events); and (c) the accuracy of inner reality testing (psychological-mindedness and awareness of inner states).

2. *Judgment*: The components are (a) awareness of appropriateness of, and likely consequences of, intended behavior (anticipation of probable dangers, legal culpabilities and social censure, or disapproval); and (b) extent of manifest behavior as a reflection of the awareness of these likely consequences.

3. *Sense of Reality of the World and of the Self*: The components are (a) the extent to which external events are experienced as real and as being embedded in a familiar context (degree of derealization, *déjà vu*, trancelike states); (b) the extent to which the body (or parts of it) and its functioning and one's behavior are experienced as familiar, unobtrusive, and as belonging to (or emanating from) the individual; (c) the degree to which the person has developed individuality, uniqueness, and a sense of self and self-esteem; and (d) the degree to which the person's self-representations are separated from his object representations.

4. *Regulation and Control of Drives, Affects, and Impulses*: The components are (a) the directness of impulse expression (ranging from primitive acting-out through neurotic acting-out to relatively indirect forms of behavioral expression); and (b) the effectiveness of delay and control, the degree of frustration tolerance, and the extent to which drive derivatives are channeled through ideation, affective expression, and manifest behavior.

5. *Object (or Interpersonal) Relationships*: The com-

ponents are (a) the degree and kind of relatedness to others and investment in them (taking account of withdrawal trends, narcissistic self-concern, narcissistic object choice, or mutuality); (b) the extent to which present relationships are adaptively or maladaptively influenced by, or patterned on, older ones, and serve present, mature aims rather than past, immature ones; (c) the degree to which the person perceives others as separate entities rather than as extensions of himself; and (d) the extent to which he can maintain object constancy (i.e., sustain relationships over long periods of time and tolerate both the physical absence of the object, and frustration, anxiety, and hostility related to the object).

6. *Thought Processes*: The components are (a) the adequacy of processes that adaptively guide and sustain thought (attention, concentration, anticipation, concept formation, memory, and language); and (b) the extent of relative primary-secondary process influences on thought (degree to which thinking is unrealistic, illogical, and/or loose).

7. *Adaptive Regression in the Service of the Ego*: The components are (a) relaxation of perceptual and conceptual acuity and other ego controls with a concomitant increase in awareness of previously preconscious and unconscious contents (first phase of an oscillating process); and (b) induction of new configurations that increase adaptive potentials as a result of creative integrations (second phase of the oscillating process).

8. *Defensive Functioning*: The components are (a) the degree to which defensive components adaptively or maladaptively affect ideation and behavior; and (b) the extent to which these defenses have succeeded or failed (degree of emergence of anxiety, depression, and/or other dysphoric affects indicating weakness of defensive operations).

9. *Stimulus Barrier*: The components are (a) a threshold for, sensitivity to, or awareness of stimuli impinging on various sensory modalities (primarily external, but including pain); and (b) the nature of response to var-

ious levels of sensory stimulation in terms of the extent of disorganization, avoidance, withdrawal, or active coping mechanisms employed to deal with them.

10. *Autonomous Functioning*: The components are (a) degree of freedom from impairment of apparatuses of primary autonomy (functional disturbances of sight, hearing, intention, language, memory, learning, or motor function); and (b) degree of, or freedom from, impairment of secondary autonomy (disturbances in habit patterns, learned complex skills, work routines, hobbies, and interests).

11. *Synthetic-Integration Functioning*: The components are (a) degree of reconciliation or integration of discrepant or potentially contradictory attitudes, values, affects, behavior, and self-representations; and (b) degree of active relating together and integrating of psychic and behavioral events, whether contradictory or not.

12. *Mastery-Competence*: The components are (a) extent of competence, that is, the person's performance in relation to his existing capacity to interact with and master his environment; and (b) extent of sense of competence, that is, the person's expectation of success or the subjective side of actual performance (how well he believes he can do).

Rating Ego Functions

Drawing on psychoanalytic theory and practice, a coding manual was constructed. For each ego function, the observer uses a scale running from 1 (poor or minimal functioning) to 13 (optimal functioning). (An alternative form used 1–7.) Of course, extremes rarely exist in reality, so 1s and 13s are rarely used. The number 11 represents the "average" functioning, defined by absence of significant pathology but short of optimal functioning.

The manual was written so that detailed descriptions could be used for alternate points on the scale (3, 5, 7, 9, 11, and 13). Recall that each function was divided into components. In order to improve the precision of the assessment, each of the components was rated individually. For example, in assessing the ego function of reality testing, the first component is "distinction between inner and outer stimuli." Here are a few representative anchor points used in scoring it. (I have left out the descriptions for points 3, 7, and 11.)

> *Point 1:* Hallucinations and delusions pervade. Minimal ability to distinguish events occurring in dreams from those occurring in waking life, and inability to distinguish among idea, image, and hallucination. Perceptual experience is grossly disturbed (e.g., moving things look still and vice versa).
>
> *Point 5:* Illusions are more likely to be found than hallucinations. Patient may be aware of seeing and hearing things that are not there but knows that others do not see or hear them.
>
> *Point 9:* Confusion about inner and outer states occurs mainly on awakening, going to sleep, or under severe stress.
>
> *Point 13:* Clear awareness of whether events occurred in dreams or waking life. Correct identification of the source of cognitive and/or perceptual content as being idea or image, and accurate identification of its source as internal or external. Distinction between outer and inner percepts holds up even under extreme stress. Checking perceptions against reality occurs with a very high degree of automaticity.

Using a manual made up of descriptions like these, a profile of an individual can be reliably constructed. In the next section, I will describe different ways the ratings can be done, but let me first illustrate the application of the scale.

When Mr. B. went into analysis, he craved praise and compliments from clients, employees, and the community. He worked hard to please others and enjoyed considerable success in his efforts, yet this left him unsatisfied. He felt out of place, false, and undeserving. Even mild criticism from superiors stung him and he often felt demeaned by them.

How would an ego functional assessment of Mr. B. proceed? Consider ego function number 3, labeled "sense of reality of the world and of the self." Each of the 13 points associated with the ego function is described in detail. Point 7 says, "Role playing at identity rather than experiencing it from within. Often feels humiliated. Sometimes subject is dependent on external feedback to maintain identity." This description clearly applies to Mr. B.'s ego functioning at the beginning of analysis. Later, when Mr. B. was enjoying a period of positive transference, he was rated 2 points higher: "More . . . stable identity, self-image, and self-esteem noted here. There are signs of independence, sense of self with a moderately good sense of inner identity, continuity, and internalized self-representation."

Consider a contrasting example. Ms. C. experienced a suicidal crisis, during which she swallowed 200 mg of secobarbital on the anniversary of her mother's death. Inside herself, she felt empty. She began to feel a global floating feeling of being inside the body of her mother. Simultaneously, those important to her seemed far away, like dwarfs or small statues. Before she took the pills, she had gone to her parents' apartment. Although she was familiar with it, everything seemed bizarrely transformed. The medication took effect and she had a dream fantasy that by ingesting the whole bottle of secobarbital she might blend and merge with her mother, allowing each to be inside the other's body. Again and again, she looked in the mirror, only to see her mother's face there.

How would the clearly more disturbed ego functioning of Ms. C. be rated? If we again turn to ego function number 3, labeled "sense of reality of the world and of the self," we find this description at point 1: "Surrounding people and things feel unreal, changed in appearance, as though they weren't there—very slight environmental changes may produce strange sensations. There may be oceanic feelings of nothingness, feeling dead, inanimate, selfless. Parts of the body feel unreal . . . feeling literally or physically empty inside . . . may experience states of extreme fusion or merging with others, suggesting near-total loss of boundaries between the self and the outside world. At this stop, body boundaries may be extremely fluid and vulnerable."

It seems this nightmarish episode is one of those unusual instances that qualify for an extreme rating of 1.

Naturally, Ms. C. was not always this disturbed. Her rating of 1 on this component of an ego function was a snapshot at a given moment in time. For this reason, it is often useful to secure ratings more than one time. This method allows the clinician or researcher to quantify changes, producing a fluid profile of the individual.

The Research Project

For the reader who wants to know more about the use of ego function assessment, I recommend Bellak, Hurvich, and Gediman (1973), which describes in detail the conceptual background of the instrument, as well as its construction and validation on groups of normals, neurotics, and schizophrenics; and Bellak and Goldsmith's (1984) *The Broad Scope of Ego Function Assessment*. In this section, I will mention only a few aspects of the study that are of interest to the general reader.

Subjects were recruited from local hospital wards, psychotherapy clinics, and hospital administrative personnel. They were matched as closely as possible for IQ, age, education, and socioeconomic status. Schizophrenic subjects were between 20 and 45 years old, had been diagnosed by two different psychiatrists not connected with the project (and unfamiliar with ego functional assessment), and with no evidence of brain syndromes, alcoholism, the use of hard drugs, or long-term hospitalization (over one year). Volunteer neurotics and normals were recruited with a memorandum inviting participation.

Subjects were screened. If admitted to the study, they were interviewed according to the structured interview manual by an interviewer who was a psychoanalyst, psychoanalytically oriented psychotherapist, or graduate student. Raters were given rating forms, which required that they write down the primary information that formed the basis of the rating and any secondary inferences they might make.

Since neither the interviewers nor the raters took part in the selection of subjects, the chances were lessened that they knew whether the subject was from the schizophrenic, neurotic, or normal group. Nevertheless, perfect double-blind conditions were spoiled by the occasional remark a schizophrenic subject might make about life on the ward or a frank psychotic episode.

An obvious requirement of an ego function assessment is that it classify more disturbed persons as having lower functioning. Although there was some expected overlap in the distribution of normal, neurotic, and schizophrenic subjects, significant differences were found on ratings. (The mean for normals was 9.08; for neurotics, 7.42; and for schizophrenics, 5.86.) Also, reasonable reliability is necessary. Using our specially designed manual, which can be found in the appendix of Bellak, Hurvich, and Gediman (1973), interrater reliability between two judges who formally evaluated a subject ranged from 0.61 for the ego function labeled "stimulus barrier" to 0.88 for "autonomous functioning," with a mean correlation of 0.77. (However, I have also found that ratings based on everyday psychotherapy sessions allow for an interrater reliability of 0.72, indicating the clinical usefulness of the assessment.)

Ego Function Assessment and Therapeutic Response

Many important treatment decisions can be facilitated by ego functional assessment.

Crisis Intervention

In crisis intervention, an ego function assessment can allow the clinician to judge which functions are intact and can be relied on to support the patient prior to a hospitalization. Poor impulse control might indicate immediate use of medications. Poor synthetic-integrative functioning might indicate that the patient is not ready for insight-oriented therapy.

Psychopharmacology

Considerable data have by now been collected that allow us to anticipate that some medicines given for psychiatric illnesses will affect specific target symptoms. Since these symptoms can often be understood as manifestations of defects in ego function, the physician can be guided in his prescription practices. Similarly, in monitoring treatment with psychotropic medication, a preliminary ego functional assessment provides a valuable baseline for evaluating the effectiveness of various medicines. Obviously, an assessment should be repeated at regular intervals.

Predicting Analyzability

If an analyst is considering whether a patient should undertake an analysis, the analyst might use the list of ego functions as a checklist, to reason as follows:

1. *Reality testing* requires a reasonable ability to distinguish inner and outer stimuli. Without this ability, the patient's response to current situations may be too heavily determined by infantile fantasies. An unmanageable transference may develop, or the patient may be expected to act out.
2. *Judgment* is required for the patient to set analytic goals and appreciate the long-term financial and practical demands of the treatment.
3. Patients with significant impairments in their *sense of reality* are at risk for a regressive refusion with the analyst, which could give rise to a transference psychosis.

4. *The regulation of drives* is important not only because poor regulation may predict acting out but also because overtly gratifying symptomatology combined with deficient drive regulation produces an extremely difficult-to-treat set of problems. (Many of today's crack abusers may fall into this category.)
5. Without some capacity for *object relations,* no tie with the analyst can develop. Even moderate disturbances can leave the patient especially prone to problems with silences, breaks, and so on.
6. *Free association*—a primary tool of analytic work—requires sufficiently intact thought processes to move back and forth between primary and secondary process material.
7. Without abilities to suspend secondary processes, allowing an *adaptive regression in the service of the ego,* and also to reverse the regression in order to utilize the new perceptions it allows, meaningful insight cannot be developed.
8. *Defensive functioning* must provide an adequate buffer against emergent affect so that the patient is not overwhelmed, but it must not be too rigid.
9. The patient's *stimulus barrier* must allow screening out of external stimuli so that he can turn inward.
10. Prior to the analysis, the patient needs to have developed *autonomous functioning* (e.g., such as memory, language, attention, used in the analytic work) and habits, skills, and patterns that support the practical necessities of the work.
11. Although the analyst supports the *synthetic-integrative functioning* of the patient, if the patient is to utilize the analytic insight he must eventually supply the greater part of this for himself.
12. *Mastery-competence* is required if the patient is to avoid stagnation. I have found that patients with strong passive or masochistic wishes present problems in analysis.

The Broad Scope of Ego Function Assessment

Contemporary Psychiatry

One frequently hears the complaint that psychiatrists have so many disagreements that they find it hard to have useful conversations with each other. One advantage I see to ego function assessment is that it can serve as a bridge between psychodynamic and descriptive psychiatry. Caregivers of all persuasions will naturally be interested in how well the patient's ego functions, for this information allows predictions to be made about dangerousness, independent living, responses to treatment, and the like.

Psychological Testing

An ambiguity that has dogged the use of popular psychological tests (such as the Rorschach, Thematic Apperception Test, and Children's Apperception Test) is the uncertainty about how test findings relate to primary clinical data. In a series of studies, I have found ego function assessment useful with psychological testing. In fact, the graphic form used to provide a profile of ego functioning can easily be used to summarize psychological test results.

Third-Party Payments

As I mention in the last section of Chapter Eight, the changing economic environment of psychiatric and psychotherapeutic work now puts a premium on objective ways of demonstrating that treatment is effective (and that third-party payers are getting results for their money). If change is to be demonstrated, there must be comparability among the results of evaluations.

Any assessment that takes place should have clear consequences for treatment planning. If a patient who is experiencing an acute psychotic episode with impaired reality testing, thought processes, and judgment also has a history of overall high levels of ego functioning with marked capacities for mastery and competence, treatment would sensibly combine an inpatient setting with intensive psychotherapy, since his prognosis is relatively good. If, on the other hand, a similarly ill patient has a history of low levels of ego functioning from an early age, with poor object relations and little strength in mastery-competence, he might be better treated with supportive psychotherapy and psychopharmacology.

When justifying the duration of a treatment, consideration of symptomatic relief is not enough. The individual's overall ability to function must also be measured.

Prevention

As evidence accumulates that serious psychiatric illness often has a basis in various types of brain dysfunction, it becomes important to understand the response of the personality to these dysfunctions. Prophylactic treatment may be usefully designed to support intact ego structures and to address the specific ego site where brain dysfunctions reduce ego functioning.

GRAPHIC REPRESENTATION

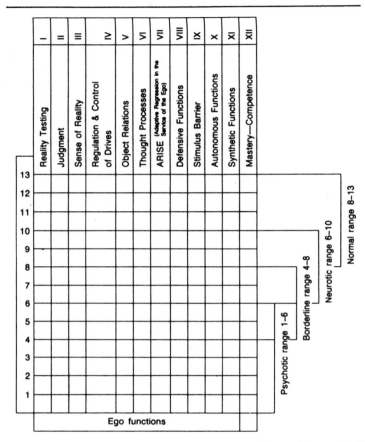

Reprinted by permission of John Wiley & Sons. From: Bellak, Hurvich, & Gediman, *Ego Functions in Schizophrenics, Neurotics, and Normals,* 1973, New York.

CHAPTER SEVEN

Philosophy and Psychoanalysis

Bad Feelings and Suspicion

Philosopher Sidney Hook, who organized an important conference on philosophy and psychoanalysis in 1958, used to describe what he felt to be his long-suffering quest for a straight answer from psychoanalysts. He told how, starting in 1919, he began to ask psychoanalysts he met the same question he would eventually ask in 1958: What evidence, if any, would indicate that, in a given instance, a child did not have an oedipus complex? Hook said the conference was memorable to him because he obtained from Charles Brenner and Jacob Arlow what he rather grudgingly called "something of an intelligible answer to my question" (Hook, 1959, p. 216). Having finally gotten what he asked for, this typically rigorous philosophical thinker proceeded to tear into the reply with such eagerness that he committed some rather elementary logical errors.

Unfortunately, Hook's feelings have been widely shared by many philosophers who have addressed psychoanalysts. For much of the troubled history between these two disciplines, philosophers have felt their legitimate attempts to hold psychoanalysts to scientific standards have been met by evasions, double talk, and the defensively superior attitude the initiated take when confronted by the uninitiated. For their part, psychoanalysts have felt criticized, hounded by uncomprehending complaints, and thwarted in their own long-suffering attempts to explain patiently a complex set of relations between psychoanalytic evidence and theories—explain to impatient listeners more interested in setting traps than learning about the mind.

Familiar as I am with this sort of fruitless standoff, I have nevertheless always been a bit puzzled by it. Of course when members of one group set out to derogate the work of the other, little mutual help is to be expected. But I know for a fact that many good-faith efforts have also been made. And yet, when one thinks of the natural affinities between the two subjects, and their great potential for helping one another, I fear that even the most charitable estimate of their exchanges must conclude that the yield has been small indeed.

To simplify somewhat, most of the history of philosophical criticisms of psychoanalysis can be grouped under one of two headings, one traceable to Ludwig Wittgenstein, the other to Karl Popper. For reasons I shall make clear, let us call Wittgenstein's criticism the *cause/reason* criticism and Popper's criticism the *falsification* criticism. There was also a third, logical positivist, Viennese philosophical response, which I will discuss at the end of the chapter.

Ludwig Wittgenstein

The Wittgenstein family was widely known in Vienna. Karl Wittgenstein, the philosopher's father, was an engineer and successful businessman whose innovations had helped revive the late-blooming Austrian iron industry. One could read his opinions on economic matters of the day in the city's main newspaper, the *Neue Freie Presse*. His wife and several of their children were accomplished musicians. The family's great wealth enabled them to patronize the city's arts and to create a highly cultured home, visited by Gustav Mahler, Bruno Walter, Johannes Brahms, Pablo Casals, and others. The philosopher's brother, Paul, was a well-known concert pianist, despite the fact that he had lost an arm in the First World War. There is a well-known portrait of his youngest sister, Margarete, by the painter Gustav Klimt.

The philosopher's early encounters with Freud's writings may have been at Margarete's prompting, for she knew Freud personally and assisted Marie Bonaparte when the Anschluss made it necessary for her to leave Austria for England. In his classes at Cambridge, Wittgenstein described a case in which she mentioned to Freud a topic of common interest (some paintings they had seen), and then reported back to her brother Freud's interpretation (1980, p. 4). She may also have given her brother more than a textbook acquaintance with psychoanalytic methods, for, it was said that, like the family's houseguest Gustav Mahler, Margarete also sought psychoanalytic help for emotional problems.

Like his father Karl, Wittgenstein had a flair for technical matters; both studied engineering. After he graduated from the *Realgymnasium,* Ludwig went first to the Technical University in Berlin, and then to the University of Manchester where, as a research student, he worked for three years on problems in aeronautics. His interest in certain mathematical problems led him to search out the advice of well-known logicians such as Bertrand Russell and Gottlieb Frege and, ultimately, to his career in philosophy.

It seems to me that, in his philosophy, as in his life, Wittgenstein was a man divided: divided between Cambridge, where he taught and eventually rose to a professorship, and Vienna, to which he continued to return at regular intervals; divided between his early involvement in rather abstract problems of logic, culminating in his *Tractatus Logico-Philosophicus* (1922), which he considered to have effectively solved philosophical problems, and his later involvement with the way ordinary people use expressions, found in his *Philosophical Investigations* (1953); and, finally, divided between his admiration for technical precision and the otherworldly, almost mystical, longing sensed in certain passages of his work.

One can see this divided mind even in Wittgenstein's predominantly negative evaluation of psychoanalysis. A notebook entry from 1946, for example, tries to contain his admiration within a parenthesis: "Freud's fanciful pseudo-explanations (precisely because they are so brilliant) perform a disservice" (1980, p. 55).

His main objection to psychoanalysis seems to have been that it involved what he labeled "a muddle between a cause and a reason" (1980, p. 10). If we want to talk about the *reason* someone did something, Wittgenstein said, then agreement plays a crucial role. But if the *cause* of an action is at issue, experiments are needed. His main concern was seemingly to oppose the scientific claims of psychoanalysis. Sometimes he complains that psychoanalytic ideas are pre-scientific ("Freud is constantly claiming to be scientific. But what he gives is *speculation*—something prior even to the formation of any hypothesis," (1982, p. 3)). At other times, he seems to doubt that they are "pre-" anything; they are more like an aesthetic idea than an early phase of science. ("What Freud says about the subconscious sounds like science, but in fact it is just a means of representation. . . . The display of elements in a dream is a display of similes. As in aesthetics, things are placed side by side so as to exhibit certain features" [1982, p. 10].)

These and other criticisms of psychoanalysis set the tone for a generation of British philosophers who condemned it for its "conceptual confusions"; yet Wittgenstein himself was by no means hostile to Freud in an unqualified way. Once, for example, after having arranged for the financial aid needed for a student he had persuaded to leave philosophy for medicine (and eventually psychiatry), Wittgenstein sent the student (M. O'C. Drury) a gift of Freud's *Interpretation of Dreams,* explaining that when he first read it, he thought to himself, "Here, at last, is a psychologist with something to say" (Drury, 1984, p. 136). Interestingly, Wittgenstein's ambivalence appears elsewhere in his letter to the former student, when he asks Drury to make inquiries at his medical school because he (Wittgenstein) was considering leaving philosophy to train as a psychiatrist.

Even though he never actually took this step, he frequently asked his student to describe cases to him and once arranged for permission to interview psychiatric patients at the hospital where Drury practiced.

Guesswork about the feelings of a stranger is always risky, but Wittgenstein seems to have felt some of the same curiosity about the mind and mental illness that I felt so many years ago. If so, why did he not feel the same attraction to psychoanalysis? There are passages in Wittgenstein's works that certainly suggest he believed that the Freudian elements he found nonscientific were nevertheless profound. There is evidence he worried that the technical orientation of science and its tendency to view problems as something to be fixed would, when directed toward the mind, lead to a tinkering, meddlesome attitude. ("Don't play with what lies deepest in another person," he recorded in his notebook at one point [1980, p. 23]. And he once told Drury that analysis could be a "dangerous procedure" and that he knew of a case where it did "infinite harm.") It sounds as if Wittgenstein felt a constitutional wariness and distaste for the intrusions of examining private matters with the lens of an impersonal, almost public, practice like science.

Of course, speculations about Wittgenstein's attitudes do not bear on the validity of his views. And he may have held only the conceptual objections I summarized earlier. After all, there is a long tradition of opposing scientific examination of the mental life, dating at least as far back as Immanuel Kant.

Causes, Reasons, and Little Red Books

Regardless of any personal attitudes that may have affected Wittgenstein's views of psychoanalysis, his objections were soon taken up by a generation of British philosophers. This new generation of Wittgensteinians seems to lack entirely the deep unworldly elements so characteristic of Wittgenstein.

Wittgenstein's way of philosophizing on a variety of topics took English-speaking universities by storm. Whether the topic was perception, ethics, or dreams, the new philosophers copied Wittgenstein's practice of examining closely the implicit logic of the various concepts involved in a topic area. However, subtle changes in tone crept in as Wittgenstein's approach was combined with a native British philosophy of ordinary language. The procedure that resulted consisted of asking how working scientists, lawyers, or other experts used certain crucial terms, trying to learn what was involved in their arguments. Often, however, the true purpose was not so much to learn as to give a grade to the expert uses, measuring them not by the demands of science but by the yardstick of commonsense notions of causality, mind, action, or whatever. It was assumed that when experts tried to use terms in ways that were significantly at odds with the ordinary uses, they became confused.

Gone, for the most part, was the sort of sincere admiration embodied in Wittgenstein's remark that Freud was a psychologist "with something to say." Indeed, it was highly characteristic of the new approach to show little interest in what Freud actually had to say, concentrating instead on the form Freud used in arranging his arguments and theories. Hostile writers viewed psychoanalysis as a hopelessly confused jumble of ideas. Even the friendly writers were condescending, charitably offering to tidy things up for Freud, who was assumed to have innocently, if perhaps absentmindedly, created a variety of conceptual monstrosities. A few took Freud's contribution seriously and offered suggestions intended to provide genuine help in formulating psychoanalytic propositions.

Articles appeared in the British journal *Analysis* and in a series of monographs called *Studies in Philosophical Psychology* published by Routledge & Kegan Paul, sometimes called the "little red books" because they were bound in red. One discussion in *Analysis* began with Toulmin (1948), who argued that psychoanalytic propositions are different from ordinary first-person explanations of behavior, when a person gives his reason for an action ("I'm doing this because . . ."), different from reported explanations of behavior ("He did it because . . ."), and different from causal explanations, when a person is said to act under the influence of forces (because, for example, he was given an injection of cocaine). First-person explanations, Toulmin said, were reports that could neither be proved nor disproved. Reported explanations can be mistaken but they can be verified by first person reports. Causal explanations are proved or disproved by observations.

Flew (1949, 1956) took another tact, arguing that Freudian practice contradicted Freudian theory. Freudian practice was concerned with motives, intentions, and meanings, whereas the theory was concerned with antecedent causes. (This was a line later taken up by George Klein, when he argued for an independent clinical theory.) Flew came to think that psychoanalysis supported the ordinary way of speaking about motives, about why people act as they do. Psychoanalysis went beyond ordinary descriptions of motives, only that it said some motives were unconscious. From this point of view, the scientific claims of psychoanalysis—the theory of the unconscious causes that determine motives—was illegitimate. Freud's keen clinical eye was betrayed by his scientific ambitions.

In *The Concept of Motivation* (1958), R. S. Peters tried to describe psychoanalysis as a drama of Freud's promising insight betrayed by inappropriate ambitions. Early on, Peters said, Freud was content to confine his work to explaining only those cases when a thought, feeling, or action makes no sense or when the reason given for it is very unconvincing. So it is only when, for instance, the obsessive fails to be convinced by dozens of confirmations that he turned off the gas, that we are entitled to ask what causes him to be blind to the evidence of his senses, or only when the teacher (plausibly) recommends spanking so regularly that it becomes implausible, that we are entitled to look for unconscious sadism. As long as an action is sensible, there is really no point in looking for unconscious causes. However, according to Peters, Freud grew restless and expanded the scope of his theory in a philosophically unsound way. The result was a back-and-forth movement between descriptions of causes of action and descriptions of motives for action.

Peters evidently had difficulty making up his mind about Freud. He submitted his manuscript to Freud's follower, Ernest Jones, who naturally took issue with many of Peters's criticisms, as well as some of his factual statements. These responses appear in a series of footnotes, so the reader first sees Peters's description of Freud, and then Jones's warning not to accept what Peters says. Similarly, after having followed the Wittgenstein tradition of taking Freud to task for failing to fit neatly into the cause/reason scheme, Peters praises Freud's "lasting contribution," which was to show "that neither the rule-following purposive model nor the mechanical model of explanation are really adequate for conceptualizing his revolutionary insights" (1958, p. 94).

The same year the Peters book came out, the author of another book in the same series chided his fellow philosophers for not recognizing how thoroughgoing was the conceptual confusion in Freud. In *The Unconscious* (1958), A. C. MacIntyre joined in the chorus that said Freud "tries to treat unconscious motives both as purposes and as causes. This is simply a confusion" (p. 60). MacIntyre went further, however, pointing out that it did no good to protect Freud's reputation by attributing to him a good, clinical theory (expressed in the sort of reason-giving, motivational language that would later be favored by British philosophers) alongside his bad, mistaken theoretical system (expressed in a language of causes and forces). In both Freud's theory making and his clinical reports, MacIntyre claimed, Freud confused a language of causes and a language of motives—though, in fairness, MacIntyre noted that, in the latter case, the "confusion [is] rooted in the realities of the therapeutic situation" (p. 66).

Other books and articles sounded similar themes during the first two decades after World War II. Although the authors clearly believed themselves to be taking issue with one another, arguing about how best to address the "conceptual confusions" in Freud, the observer in the 1990s is struck by an agreement of both style and substance. Freud is first praised for his "innovations" or his "genius," and then given a low grade based on his failure to distinguish properly *causes* of a *behavior* from reasons for it. (Never mind, of course, that the same journals and publications series show that even philosophers within this fairly homogeneous school could not agree among themselves what this distinction meant.)

Some of these criticisms of Freud were later taken to heart by theoretically minded psychoanalysts such as George Klein (1976) and, more recently, Roy Schafer (1976, 1978, 1980, 1981, 1983). Perhaps because my own philosophical attachments were closer to logical positivism, I had mixed feelings about these writings. As I wrote in an early philosophically oriented article, I believe that conceptual clarification is important and necessary for psychoanalysis. So I agreed on this methodological point. And I also saw the point these authors were making about the existence of certain tensions and conflicts between our ordinary way of speaking, which often does imply some logical differences between causes and reasons, and Freud's efforts to create a science that did not always honor these differences. Yet I did not find their complaints particularly devastating. Were not such tensions and conflicts to be expected? Didn't they accurately reflect exactly the sort of problems Freud intended to raise when he chose to describe the mental life as determined, fragmented, and caught in the play of forces?

Sometime in the 1960s, there was a change of attitudes among philosophers in this tradition. When MacIntyre, who had been so staunch in his opposition to Freud's confusions, was asked to write the Freud entry in the *Encyclopedia of Philosophy,* he explained that "Freud . . . wrote of unconscious motives as a kind of cause, and philosophical critics have been perhaps too hasty in supposing that he must be mistaken" (1967, p. 251). (Although MacIntyre did not say so, I think we can conclude he is confessing that he was one of those who was "perhaps too hasty.")

In the same entry, MacIntyre went further. He wrote:

Freud's discovery of the causation both of neurotic symptoms and of normal character traits fatally weakened any attempt to maintain that human behavior was essentially exempt from explanation in causal terms or that the line between responsible, rational behavior and nonresponsible irrational behavior could be drawn in terms of the applicability of the notion of cause. (1967, p. 252)

This conclusion, which had seemed to me to be an inevitable logical consequence of psychoanalysis from the time I first read Freud, was quite a dramatic concession when considered in the context of this philosophical tradition. In many articles, and in several of the little red books, the so-called incompatibility between human action and causal explanation was so often taken for granted that an author was ready to declare "no contest" once he had demonstrated that an opponent's position might call into question this assumption.

Text Appeal—Appealing to the Text

At about the same time that philosophers had cast aside the assumption of incompatibility, philosophically minded psychoanalysts began to take it up. One result of this trend has been the use of concepts such as *hermeneutics, narrative,* and *interpretation.* Although there is no necessary logical connection, these terms often appear together as elements in an argument which states that since psychoanalysis deals with human meanings, symbols, and the like, it cannot be properly understood by using causal or scientific terms.

Until the late 1960s, the case for excluding causal explanations came almost entirely from English-speaking, usually British philosophers, such as Toulmin, Flew, Peters, and MacIntyre. Some French- and German-speaking philosophers had discussed these issues, but they had little impact on the psychoanalytic community. In the last part of the sixties, this situation changed when Paul Ricoeur's *Freud and Philosophy* (1970) and Jurgen Habermas's *Knowledge and Human Interests* (1971) appeared. (These publication dates are a bit misleading. Ricoeur's book began life as the 1961 Terry lecture at Yale, and the German version of Habermas's book appeared in 1968. Many of his basic ideas on the logic of psychoanalysis were described in a 1965 address which was printed as an appendix to *Knowledge and Human Interests*.)

These new works are sometimes said to have introduced a hermeneutical perspective. Although the meaning we should give to this word is itself a matter of controversy, *hermeneutics* can be expressed, roughly, as text interpretation. (For a more extended discussion, the reader can consult the famous German exponent H. G. Gadamer [1976] or a good summary found in Seebohm [1977a, 1977b]). Its use in a psychoanalytic context is intended to suggest that the analyst's understanding of the patient resembles a reader's understanding of a text. Just as a reader considers a word in the context of a sentence, a sentence in the context of a paragraph, a whole book in the context of a genre, and so on, the analyst applies a similar method in trying to make sense of what the patient has to say. Sometimes the term *hermeneutics* is also meant to imply an equation between the reader and the analyst: Neither is concerned with causes or with asking questions that could be solved by experiments. Spence (1982, 1983, 1986), for example, has applied hermeneutical ideas in describing his view of the psychoanalytic process.

(Technically speaking, it may not be correct to characterize Ricoeur and Habermas as offering hermeneutic versions of psychoanalysis. Ricoeur has emphasized that, like all analogies, the analogy between reader and text, and psychoanalyst and patient, breaks down because, as he acknowledges, psychoanalysis is a method of investigation as well as a clinical enterprise. And Habermas has pointed out why, even though psychoanalysis is hermeneutical, it differs from other hermeneutical approaches. As for myself, I refer the reader back to Chapter One and the importance of continuity and causality in psychoanalysis as a science that permits prediction and postdiction.)

In the 1960s, psychoanalysts themselves began to assimilate pieces of these arguments. In the English-speaking tradition, George Klein (1976), a promising theorist and researcher, argued that clinical psychoanalytic theory was and ought to be a separate enterprise from the metapsychological or theoretical psychoanalytic theory. The former was concerned with the meaningful data of sessions and expressed in the language of purpose, intentions, and so on; the latter was concerned with functional systems and expressed in the language of energy, mechanics, and the like. In a volume prepared in memory of Klein (who had died young), Merton Gill and Philip Holzman elaborated on his argument. Gill pleaded for psychoanalysts to disentangle purely psychological clinical propositions from the physicalist, mechanistic language of the metapsychology. And Holzman showed how, among psychoanalysts, the metapsychology had begun to serve as a cryptosomatic theory, immune to modification by sound physical (and sometimes nonpsychoanalytic) research, yet also resistant to psychological clinical data, which could not be expressed in mechanistic terms.

More recently, Schafer has combined rejection of causal explanation with a hermeneutical interest to produce a narrative version of psychoanalysis. The patient's productions (like the analyst's guiding theories) are seen as narratives. In neither case is a traditional scientific concern for uncovering the truth emphasized; instead, the focus is on how all versions implicitly sketch a portrait of patient, analyst, and their work. It is desirable, Schafer suggests, for analysts to be aware of how these implicit images often describe the patient as passive, acted on by forces.

Karl Popper

Though less wealthy than the Wittgenstein family, the family of the philosopher Sir Karl Popper belonged to the solid professional class that played an important role in the life of the city. The Popper family was distantly related to Josef Popper-Lynkeus, a philosopher and scientist who was well known at that time, although he is not widely remembered today. The philosopher's father, like his two uncles, was a doctor of law of the University. He had been a partner of the last liberal Burgomaster of Vienna, Dr. Carl Grubl. His mother was from the Schiff family, who played an active part in the musical world of the city.

The reader can glean a basic impression of the small world of Viennese intellectual community from the fact that, just as in my case and in the case of Ludwig Wittgenstein, there was a personal connection to the Freud family. Freud's sister, Rosa Graf, the great-aunt of W. Ernst Halberstadt Freud, sometimes vacationed with Popper's parents. In his autobiography, *Unended Quest* (1974), which I have used as a source, the philosopher recalled a visit during World War I from Freud's nephew, Hermann Graf; it was his last leave before going to the front, where he met his death. Popper mentions no further connections to the Freud family.

Since Popper's denunciation of psychoanalysis is one of the most frequently cited, one might expect a detailed, exhaustive argument. Instead, what one finds is a mostly autobiographical account in which psychoanalysis, marxism, and Adlerian psychology are presented as examples of what a scientific theory must avoid.

Popper formed his views on psychoanalysis when he was 17 years old. He had recently departed secondary school without graduating, taking classes as a nonmatriculated student at the University, intent on self-education. Like many of those faced with the chaos and hardship following the breakdown of the Austrian Empire at the close of World War I, Popper drifted briefly into communism. Not long after he became a confirmed marxist, an incident occurred in which the authorities opened fire on demonstrators trying to free communists held by the police. Some communists had pressed for the violent confrontation; Popper felt guilty because he believed that, as a marxist, he was committed to an intensification of the class struggle that might legitimate such confrontations. He began to worry that he had not examined marxist ideas with sufficient skepticism.

Popper also worked for a time as a social worker. It was then that he had an occasion to present a case to Adler. He reported no similar revelation regarding psychoanalysis, but lumped together Freud with Marx and Adler in order to contrast the three with Einstein. Unlike Einstein's theories, their theories explained too much. Their followers, once converted, found the world to be filled with confirmations; it was necessary, however, to find refutations. To get these, scientists had to make risky predictions, specifying what would falsify a theory, as with Einstein's specific descriptions of astronomical findings, tested during an eclipse in May 1919. Thus Popper concluded that because psychoanalysis was so hard to refute, it should not be considered a fully scientific discipline.

Falsification and Standards of Science

The charge that psychoanalysis could not be falsified—a concept close to the more commonly used one of testing the null hypothesis—surfaced again and again. Popper, especially, chose the hypothesis of the oedipus complex for this purpose. Since Freud had said that it was omnipresent, Popper felt that the null hypothesis could not be tested. Leaving the doubtful merits of this argument, there are literally dozens (if not hundreds) of psychoanalytic hypotheses that can be not only verified but also falsified (e.g., those mentioned in Chapter Four).

Something like this sentiment must have been behind Sidney Hook's question about the oedipus complex mentioned earlier in this chapter, dating from the March 1958 Symposium on Psychoanalysis, Scientific Method, and Philosophy at New York University's Institute of Philosophy. Hook described the meeting as the "first time in the United States that a distinguished group of psychoanalysts has met with a distinguished philosophers of science in a free, critical interchange of views on the scientific status of psychoanalysis" (1959, p. xiii). The published proceedings of the symposium make clear how prominent the concern about falsification was. During the conference, the psychoanalyst Heinz Hartmann laid out a view of psychoanalysis as a scientific theory and the philosopher Ernest Nagel responded with methodological and logical criticisms.

Much of Hartmann's career had been dedicated to this topic; his piece showed his concern with the functional definitions. He also included material on potentially valuable new types of evidence that might improve psychoanalytic science, including contemporary studies I was conducting. (I recorded sessions that were then presented to other analysts, who were asked to make predictions about subsequent sessions. These are discussed in Chapter Eight.) For his part, Nagel worried that there might be no way of choosing among alternative, competing interpretations, all equally coherent, of the same clinical data. Hartmann had said that the psychoanalyst could base his choice on either the outcome of predictions made, or on laws based on experience with other patients. Nagel doubted these alternatives were adequate; the link between a given interpretation and a predicted change in the patient was not logically strict enough, and the so-called laws had been established without proper controls. The result was that too many things might be "true" at once.

The published proceedings contain not only the papers of the presenters but also "Discussion, Criticism, and Contributions by Other Participants" which were submitted to the editor after the sessions were over. It is in this section that Hook's request appeared for a specification of evidence that might prove the absence of an oedipal complex. Although Hook said he "received something of an intelligible answer" from Drs. Charles Brenner and Jacob Arlow, other analysts took issue with his request for a specification of evidence. Dr. Lawrence Kubie said it was not proper to ask for overt behavioral evidence since the question at issue concerned states or processes that are not conscious. In a one-page attack on Kubie, another philosopher charged that by making the hypothesis of the oedipus complex independent of overt behavior, "Dr. Kubie's conception makes it *irrelevant* to the explanation of observable human behavior," and went on to compare Kubie's protective maneuver to an "exact analogue" in the reasoning of some of those who opposed the special theory of relativity in physics (1959, p. 225).

The tenor of the times can be expressed in a few general themes. Philosophers in this tradition accused psychoanalysis of making things too easy on itself when it comes to evidence. It was not that it lacked support; everyone conceded that psychoanalysis could cite evidence. Rather, theories and hypotheses needed careful arrangement so that they could be proved wrong if they failed to correspond to the facts. Only when this task had been done could psychoanalysis expect the advanced evolution characteristic of the development of the physical sciences.

It would be a mistake, however, to overlook certain differences among the philosophers in this tradition. For example, although Grünbaum was at that time working on logical questions about space and time in physics, he has more recently devoted himself to a much more detailed discussion of psychoanalysis in which he takes issue with Popper. In a series of articles, and in his widely discussed book, *The Foundations of Psychoanalysis: A Philosophical Critique* (1984), Adolf Grünbaum suggested that there may have been less than meets the eye to Popper's position.

According to Grünbaum, Popper was arguing with a straw man of his own creation. Popper indicted a very simple-minded view, which Grünbaum labels "enumerative inductivism." This view says that as one collects more and more confirmations of a theory, the theory becomes stronger and stronger. Popper was, of course, correct to point out that this road could easily lead to mischief. What was needed was what Grünbaum labels the "declared consequence restriction." This restriction states that if one wants to count an event as evidence in favor of a theory because it is a consequence of the theory, one is not permitted to know in advance if the event actually occurred or not. As long as one has declared in advance that such-and-such is a consequence of a theory, then when such-and-such occurs, it can count for the theory. Psychoanalysis, Grünbaum concluded, could be properly defended against Popper's charge because it makes possible predictions of this type.

Grünbaum was ready with a charge of his own, however, that data from the psychoanalytic session are so hopelessly contaminated that they cannot be used to support psychoanalytic propositions. Despite the attention Grünbaum's book has received, my impression is that on the whole, philosophers of science are less inclined to view psychoanalysis in this way. Many factors may be responsible; within philosophy of science, there is more interest today in how sciences actually develop and less interest in drawing a line between what is and is not scientific. Thus philosophers are less inclined to pass judgment than before. Also, it may be that psychoanalysis seems less novel than it did 30 or 40 years ago when these controversies raged. Battles between philosophers and scientists over how research on the mind should proceed are probably more likely to be found in debates about so-called artificial intelligence, intentional systems, and cognitive neuroscience. Sometimes disputes end (or at least taper off) without being resolved. It may be that the attention of philosophers who want to argue about scientific standards has moved on to other matters, even as philosophers interested in interpretation have turned to psychoanalysis.

A Matter of Attitude

At the beginning of this chapter, I said I would mention a third way in which philosophers have responded to psychoanalysis. This third way can also be traced to Vienna.

Near the end of Hook's (1959) *Psychoanalysis, Scientif-*

ic Method, and Philosophy, one finds a brief comment by the physicist/philosopher Philipp Frank. In it, this original member of the scientifically minded Vienna Circle tried to set the record straight about the relation between psychoanalysis and the philosophical movement called logical positivism. Frank described how the doctrines of logical positivism had come to be seen as uncompromising gatekeepers, blocking entry into science of any but the most logically strict theories—those whose terms have met rigorous semantic standards and proven themselves to be meaningful.

Frank began by reminding his audience that Otto Neurath, an important member of the Vienna Circle, felt considerable enthusiasm for the new and exciting connections psychoanalysis had been able to make, despite its logical and semantic problems. Frank then recalled how logic and semantics were only two of the three parts of what he called an "indivisible trinity." The third member was the pragmatic. Unlike many of those who later claimed to represent logical positivism, its early advocates comfortably accepted that the theoretical system of axioms that organize a field cannot themselves be subject to observational tests. Instead, the logical positivist says "that one theory is more practical or convenient than another one. . . . Hence, the truth of Freudian or similar theories must not be understood otherwise than pragmatically. It may be convenient or not to accept them" (Frank, 1959, p. 311).

My impression is that there is little consensus among philosophers about how psychoanalysis ought to proceed. And the effects of this disharmony have been multiplied by the many different ways in which psychoanalysts have drawn on philosophy. The result has been a fragmentation of opinions. I cannot, of course, offer a full solution to this problem, but I do wish to recommend the logical positivist attitude as an especially helpful one. To me, it suggests that philosophers can be most effective by encouraging the use of evidence where it can be had and by urging logical clarification, yet without allowing either effort to become too dogmatic or prescriptive.

CHAPTER EIGHT

Psychoanalysis as a Form of Treatment and a Subject of Research

Throughout this book, we have discussed concepts of psychoanalysis as a general psychology. All of these concepts are, of course, interrelated with and relevant to psychoanalysis as treatment. A systematic discussion of the topic of psychoanalysis as therapy is in order.

My underlying views on psychoanalysis as therapy are learning theory and perceptual theory, especially that of *Gestalt* psychology. In this vein, the patient comes to us as an integration of his past experience, having "learned" to perceive people as deceitful, trusting, cruel, warm, or otherwise. In line with psychoanalytic motivational theory, some of this learning might have been more or less phase specific, and therefore more or less effective. For instance, suffering the loss of a parent in early adolescence may have more of an impact on one's conscience (because of the active conflicts and guilt feelings at that time) than at some other point in one's life. In such a case, learning as postulated by behavior psychology or cognitive psychology might also be relevant. Percept becomes structure (i.e., the structure of the superego and the ego); and the task of psychological treatment will be to change the structure into a more adaptive, less destructive one by restructuring the *gestalt.*

Psychoanalysis as a form of therapy proposes to help the patient "remember" earlier *gestalten.* These *gestalten* are often conscious only in fragments, and need to be understood in symptoms, dreams, and other productions—and by free association—as conglomerations of other *gestalten* (Bellak, 1961). With restructuring, the structures are amenable to more adaptive form—the superego might become less severe and reality testing and judgment might improve. (See Chapter Six for a discussion of ego functions.) Overall, the patient may be less troubled by distortions and painful maladaptive behavior.

Psychoanalytic technique is concerned with the optimal method of helping the patient engage in this process of restructuring. Easily enough said, but this definition is the foremost source of dissent among psychoanalysts of different persuasions. This is so primarily because psychoanalysts generally do not perceive the patient in terms of learning theory.

The crucial disagreements have traditionally revolved around the theory of transference and its role. Also in dispute is classical psychoanalysis as a treatment technique versus psychoanalytic psychotherapy, albeit also based on psychoanalytic theory.

Often because of a lack of basic understanding of the process, the dividing line between these two concepts has been a superficial indicator: The treatment technique is defined by the number of patient visits. Up to three visits a week is considered psychotherapy; any more—preferably on a couch—constitute psychoanalysis (as treatment) proper. These criteria can obscure the fact that what really matters is whether or not one operates on basic psychoanalytic concepts, such as the importance of unconscious *gestalten.*

That fact brings us to the problem of how transference

is considered as a curative factor in psychoanalysis as treatment. The classical position was that contemporary and external relationships are entirely irrelevant; what the patient projects onto the analyst from his past is relevant. The analyst concerns himself only with the analysis of the transference distortions of himself.* This conclusion disregards the fact that Freud himself had declared projection (the operative process in transference distortions) as a normal part of perception (Freud, 1913).

The analyst's behavior derives from the above viewpoint: The more classical he is, the more committed solely to the analysis of the transference, the more the analyst has to strive to be and retain himself as a *tabula rasa*—ideally a mere projection screen for the patient's sentiments. There are other analysts, however, who claim that they rarely see a transference neurosis and that their analyses seem nevertheless to be therapeutic. The fact is that one probably sees more transference and transference neurosis in the more disturbed patients, such as Freud's early ones. The healthier patient may also experience transference phenomena, but enough of his ego functions remain intact to have him aware of the distortions more of the time; at the very least he can easily be made aware of them.

In the war about transference, a major battle broke out when Franz Alexander, a Hungarian analyst later living in Chicago, started to speak of the importance of the "corrective emotional experience." What he meant was that he found it helpful to the patient to interact with him in the "here and now"—as a human being, offering warm, supportive statements when necessary, instead of making only classical interpretations. Again, seeing psychoanalytic treatment as a problem of learning renders the struggle between classical "transference neurosis" adherents and others ridiculous. The real issue is what kind of interaction, what form of unlearning and relearning is most effective

*Increasingly, the analyst concerns himself with the analysis of countertransference (i.e., of his feelings toward the patient). Thus analysis is increasingly seen as an interactive process, as is very lucidly discussed in the correspondence of Wallerstein and Gill (1991).

therapeutically in a given patient. Alexander found that patients can improve if the analyst treats them with warmth (and if psychoanalytic theory is kept in mind) rather than remaining distant and neutral.

Of course, this concept can lend itself to distortions. Jerome Frank, a prominent psychiatrist rather than a psychoanalyst, thought that nonspecific psychotherapy (i.e., psychotherapy not informed by psychoanalytic concepts) could be an effective therapy, being primarily a function of the therapist's personality and the relationship between patient and therapist.

My reply to him: If I am ill, I want warmth and fluids, but if my illness is at all serious, I also demand very specific antibiotic therapy. Carefully conceptualized, psychoanalytic treatment offers infinitely more complex unlearning and learning than a kindly relationship alone can provide.

Part of the problem of defining classical psychoanalytic treatment as distinct from psychoanalytic psychotherapy is that the concepts are concretized—treated as if there really were one process or another process "out there"—instead of it being a matter of definition. Rather than having a heated debate about *what is,* the most useful definition should be chosen. The technique most useful in classical psychoanalysis or psychoanalytic psychotherapy should be selected. (Such arguments recall discussions by the Vienna Circle and logical positivists.)

The preferred method of learning in psychoanalysis is through insight—but insight as *Gestalt* psychology defined it since Koehler's ape on Tenerife had an "aha" experience and saw the two sticks in a new *gestalt,* putting them together to make them long enough to reach the banana. Typically, by making the unconscious material preconscious, the analyst prepares the ground for the patient to have the "aha" experience himself, or to have it in response to the analyst's interpretation. However, some people are unable to have abstract insight. Adults with Attention Deficit Disorder (ADD), for instance, are often concrete thinkers and cannot utilize insight. Another form of therapy has to be found for them, albeit conceptualized in classical concepts. The moral is that the therapeutic method has to suit the patient, not the other way around.

In a basic sense, the most classical analysis also involves learning through methods other than insight. The classical psychoanalytic method of "working through" is really a form of conditioning. The patient has an insight in the session and applies it on the outside, more and more preconsciously and with increasing success. Learning by identification (with the analyst) and by introjection is also an important aspect of analytic learning. Object relations theory, as discussed (among others) by Jacobson and Kernberg, deals with introjections of *gestalt* and interaction *as gestalt* usefully, but without being aware that they are dealing with *gestalt* psychological phenomena of structuring and restructuring.

Generally speaking, the question of which therapy to use—classical analysis proper, or psychoanalytic psychotherapy, or some other form of psychotherapy—comes down to this: How this specific patient will best unlearn his maladaptive ways and change his structures* in order to find less troublesome modes of functioning.

If we keep these concepts in mind and persist in investigating the question of how psychoanalysis can be made more efficient as a technique, we may see some real progress.

Introduction to Research in Psychoanalysis

The development of research in psychoanalysis has suffered in a number of ways. Until recently, psychoanalysts, mostly physicians not trained in research and methodology, have primarily engaged in "clinical" research by listening carefully to a patient for years, usually for 50 minutes, four or five times a week. Seeing a number patients a day, they have been in a unique position to learn about mental processes in more detail and with more subtlety than anyone

---

*In *Cognitive Structures* (1957), David Rapaport spoke of structures as "processes of slow rate of change."

else. Hardly a day goes by in my own practice without some stimulating and valuable new insight, even after 40 years.

This "research," as a by-product of psychoanalysis as a therapy, has been very useful *heuristically* in formulating new hypotheses about connections between personality and life history. Yet the total number of patients that each analyst can see, which is still relatively low, has proved a major obstacle to doing anything more than satisfying each analyst's own belief that he has made a sound, valid, and reliable inference about a specific condition. The problem is similar to the one found in the story about Karl Popper's meeting with Adler. After being assured by Adler that Adler's "thousandfold experience" guaranteed his interpretation was correct, the sharp-tongued young Popper replied, "Now I suppose your experience is a thousand-and-onefold."

Case reports have been fascinating, but as far as scientific method is concerned, they are little more than anecdotal accounts. One analyst, for instance, would report his heuristic hunches based on two agoraphobic patients; others would argue the findings from their experience with another few patients. Arising from this situation is a certain amount of dogma and the wish to confirm or deny it.

In the case of agoraphobia, for instance, a verbal battle has long existed over whether its origins have preoedipal roots or only oedipal ones. Without entering into the conceptual details of the controversy, let me point out that the combatants presented mainly either/or propositions, rarely (if ever) acknowledging the possibility that in some patients oedipal factors might appear as necessary and sufficient ones for an agoraphobia, whereas in others preoedipal factors play a role.

Necessary and sufficient are key words here. Certainly physicians are acquainted with this aspect of scientific proof; for example, Koch formulated his postulates regarding tuberculosis, firmly establishing the germ theory, which holds that without tubercle bacilli there is no tuberculosis. In diagnosing tuberculosis, tubercle bacilli must be found. Thus Koch established a basic causal chain for an infectious disease. (Perhaps I should add that we now see a more complex relationship of cause and effect for tuberculosis, as well as for other diseases, in which the details are better organized through an approach like systems theory. Now that traditional medicine has begun to explore complex causality, we may find more acceptance of the sorts of operations studied by psychoanalysis.)

For the many clinically minded and medically trained psychoanalysts, scientific research has seemed a luxury; they believe that the best way to deepen understanding is to practice psychoanalysis. This mindset has been so powerful and so widespread that Freud asked: "Is the Therapy Destroying the Science?" in his discussion of professional training in *The Question of Lay Analysis* (1926b). He feared that a concentration on psychoanalysis as therapy presented a danger to the intellectual vitality of psychoanalysis (1926b, p. 256).

Was Freud's fear justified? In a limited sense, the answer is yes. Certainly the therapy has flourished more than the science. One only has to consider that the vast majority of those seeking psychoanalytic training are primarily interested in the therapeutic work. Yet Freud did not anticipate what has become clear today: In the hands of able researchers, the therapy can *be* a branch of science. Like many of his generation, Freud was enamored with the prospect of conceptually transforming more complex sciences into what were considered more basic ones. For example, he never gave up the idea that chemical interventions might substitute for psychological ones. Today, however, we no longer think it so important to make these connections. Freed of this weighty responsibility, we have been able to develop, as a largely autonomous field of study, the scientific examination of therapy. As if in exchange for our willingness to bypass the conceptual neatness of linking together various scientific fields, we are rewarded with the possibility of providing a common language in which disputes between rival psychotherapeutic factions can be investigated and resolved.

The history of the development of these studies is both

fascinating, because so much ingenuity has been required, and perplexing, because they took so long to develop. Recounting all the details of that history could take another book, so I will content myself with a few words of definition, an account of some highlights, and, finally, a few reflections. My purpose is, of course, to show that a skeptical, scientific approach is feasible; the task of reviewing this literature I leave to others.

What Makes Psychotherapy Researchable?

The term *psychotherapy* can mean so many different things. I see it as a systematic interaction between two persons—one of them a therapist, the other a patient—in which the interventions that take place use symbols. The process should follow a framework related to the personality and have as its stated goal a change in the patient. Defined in this way, psychotherapy can be researched.

I have noted with favor the development of an autonomous body of psychotherapeutic research, not tied to any one school of thought. However, I do not think psychotherapy itself should be unconnected to a theory. On the contrary, psychotherapy is a wonderfully practical arena for applying and testing the aspects of psychoanalysis I have described in previous chapters. For example, psychotherapy offers an environment for relearning. Research has supported the assumption that many psychological problems are the result of a patient's having learned to take the easy way out of frightening or painful situations, even when this makes things worse in the end. And when the patient continues to rely on these responses without checking to see if other, more productive ones might serve him better, the benign, exploratory atmosphere offered by the therapist can provide the emotional freedom and mental elbow room needed to try new responses.

I see five variables at work: the patient, the situational factors, the therapist, the therapeutic method, and time. Others have proposed other divisions, of course, but I find these useful. Ideally, to study the therapeutic method, one wants the other four factors to remain constant—but how can they? Obviously, they cannot. Therefore, one wants to control what can be controlled and, where this is not possible, use statistical methods to correct for contributions from the other factors.

A Brief Historical Background

Portions of this section draw extensively on the first chapter of *Issues in Psychotherapy Research,* by Hersen, Michelson, and Bellack (1984). The reader is referred to that work for a more in-depth narrative.

Early on, analysts at the Berlin Psychoanalytic Institute began to keep records on treatment results. Commenting on the first decade of these results, Freud wrote in his *New Introductory Lectures* (1933):

> *Its therapeutic successes give grounds neither for boasting nor for being ashamed. But statistics of that kind are in general uninstructive; the material worked upon is so heterogeneous that only very large numbers would show anything. It is wiser to examine one's individual successes. (p. 152, cited in Fisher & Greenberg, 1977, p. 276)*

Mentioned here are three elements that have played an important role in the development of psychotherapy research: studies of therapeutic outcome, case studies, and statistics.

Until very recently, Freud's negative opinion of statistical studies of outcome held sway in psychoanalytic circles. Consequently, the case study was the dominant method of research. Starting with Freud's famous cases, a genre has developed that unsystematically combines elements of a medical history with an often understated but stylish narrative and theorizing. The contributions of case studies have been substantial and there will always be a place for them.

By now, the reader can probably guess why I take issue with case studies: Too much takes place out of sight. Hypotheses are too often inexplicit or absent. Results are not audited with sufficient care. And, apart from the occasional rhetorical effort to build suspense, case studies do not say much about the many blind alleys so characteristic of both good science and good therapy. On this matter, I strongly agree with Donald Spence's conclusions that the tendency to build a convincing narrative unfortunately results in the cloaking of crucial evidence and inferences, making the scientific work of the session our "best kept secret."

In "When Interpretation Masquerades as Explanation," Donald Spence (1986) goes over one of Freud's famous cases, the Dora case. He finds Freud's compelling and dramatic narrative a bit too slick to serve as a good public (i.e., scientific) explanation of the treatment. Although the reader, like the patient, is easily caught up in the sweep of the unfolding events, he is left out of the reproducible step-by-step reasoning that one wants to find in science.

In the 1950s, psychotherapy, and the case study method in particular, was subjected to some very unfriendly criticism by those who asked the rather obvious and reasonable question: Does psychotherapy help? Of course, it was quickly discovered that although the question was obvious and reasonable, it was too simple to be very useful. It would take time before many people realized that it was more helpful to ask when, why, and how it helped, on the occasions it did help.

Early in the decade, the argument made by Hans Eysenck (1952) resounded like a challenge—a gauntlet thrown down to the psychotherapy community. Relying on large-scale statistical data collected for other purposes (e.g., hospital records and insurance claims), Eysenck said that about two-thirds of nonpsychotic psychiatric patients tend to get better even when they received little or no treatment. He then grouped together existing studies of treatment outcomes and concluded that a little under half of the patients treated with psychoanalysis are helped, and a little under two-thirds of those treated with eclectic therapies improve. So, he reasoned, psychotherapy offers little or no improvement in outcome.

The challenge was answered quickly and decisively. Many problems were found with Eysenck's argument. In his large-scale statistical analysis, "improvement" sometimes meant no more than that a person had withdrawn an insurance claim. Psychotherapeutic improvement standards are higher, so this comparison means little. Also the groups of patients compared were not very similar. And some of the groups who got better "on their own" actually got some treatment. This last point is important, because any psychotherapist knows that a single interview can be helpful, even when it is primarily devoted to diagnostic questions. This is one of those times when it is more useful to ask how even the most trivial contact with a professional might have helped.

For all the problems with the Eysenck approach, there was one sound element. He knew that if one asks "Does treatment help?" one also must take the next step and ask "Compared to what?" This second question is by no means easy to answer, however, as can be seen from the inadequacy of Eysenck's comparison with the "spontaneous remission" rate in the surveys he used.

The biggest problem—the lack of consistent standards among groups—has been dealt with in two ways. The first is to randomly assign patients to treatment or no treatment, and measure the outcome. The other is to use a sophisticated new statistical technique called meta-analysis, which uses mathematical methods to translate the findings of large numbers of studies into a common statistical language, so that they can be combined and compared.

This second approach has yielded dramatic and impressive evidence of the effectiveness of psychotherapy. Smith, Glass, and Miller (1980) reviewed 475 studies, totaling 78 different treatments, averaging 16 sessions. They found that when many measures of outcome are converted into a common statistical language, persons treated by psychotherapy show more improvement than untreated controls. Outcome, which was measured an average of four months after the start of treatment, showed that a difference between treated versus untreated was .85 of a standard deviation. In other words, 80 percent of the persons in the treated groups were better off than 50 percent of the untreated controls. Later uses of meta-analysis suggest the difference may be as much as a full standard deviation (Shapiro & Shapiro, 1982).

Curiously, the kind of psychotherapy used does not seem to make a statistically significant difference. This might seem to suggest that psychotherapies of various flavors are all pretty much the same. Yet the practitioner knows in his bones that this is not true. It is now possible to investigate and document these differences through a second major type of psychotherapy study dating from the late 1950s: the process study.

At first it was not clear how to think about the therapeutic process. In terms of the language I used earlier, was it best viewed as a therapist variable? Was it a situational variable? Or was it a therapeutic method? Carl Rogers, for example, believed that treatment effectiveness was due to the therapist's provision of warmth, empathy, unconditional positive regard, and genuineness. More importantly, he felt this was true regardless of treatment modality, and that it could be demonstrated by examination and comparison of tape recorded sessions. In this way, a concern with differences in outcome lead to consideration of process. (In the next section, I will describe my own early effort to introduce a study of process into the picture.)

As the research work of the 1950s drew to a close, an alternative to the old case study developed. Efforts had been made to understand therapeutic effect by comparing outcomes; a concern with outcomes had led to a fledgling interest in process. And, importantly, psychoanalysts were being challenged not only by unfriendly critics, who were secretly convinced psychotherapy was nonsense, but also by sympathetic advocates of alternative approaches, researchers who thought something was going on in therapy but wanted to know exactly *what*. This meant that helpful dialogue could take place. In 1958 and then again in 1961, the Division of Clinical Psychology of the American Psychological Association held conferences financed by the National Institute of Mental Health. Romantic as it may seem to be a lonely, isolated researcher, real progress usually requires a critical mass of investigators, projects, and money. These meetings were a significant step.

Once again, Eysenck (1960) entered the picture with a second attempt to make the same point: Psychotherapy is not better than no psychotherapy. In response to him, some interesting findings emerged. Data that said that, on average, therapy is not effective needed closer examination. Bergin (1963) found that this average could result from combining the results of helpful therapies with those that produced negative outcomes. As I suggested in the last section, failure to hold the therapist variable constant can lead to misinterpretation of the results.

Findings also began to accumulate that may shed some light on Eysenck's conclusions. Partly as a challenge to the authority of psychotherapists, studies compared the effectiveness of professional versus nonprofessional "therapists." Although the dispute is still a controversial one today, it was suggested that, with minimal training, nonprofessionals were as helpful as professionals (Matarazzo, 1971).

These findings have a different message for me. Think about the "untreated" controls who improved in Eysenck's studies. Undoubtedly, many of them took advantage of and were helped by the quasi-therapeutic listening skills of their friends and relatives. Once again, the limitation of an exclusive focus on outcome is clear, for the important question is how they were helped—not who helped them.

In the seventies, more attention was devoted to process research. This factor gave support to a trend that has continued into the present, a renewed interest in single case studies. Unlike the earlier case narratives that selected highlights and turning points, these "neo-case studies" put a premium on detailed attention to what happens day to day, session by session, and (lately) minute by minute. Pressure on psychoanalytic researchers to engage in such process studies came from behaviorists publishing in *Journal of Behavioral Analysis*. For example, in a single behavioral treatment, therapists would first record symptoms for a given period, then start treatment and record symptoms, then stop treatment and continue to record. Or they might alternate with another form of treatment and continue to record. This allowed them to measure what the specific effect of treatment was. The complexities of psychoanalytic psychotherapy cannot be controlled so neatly, because the effect of an analyst's words may linger or only become active when other conditions are in place. Yet many of the scientific virtues of the behaviorist design are quite possible to reproduce, such as the recording of specific, predictable effects of discrete therapeutic interventions. (See, for example, my early efforts, described in a later section.)

I have already mentioned another trend in the seventies: meta-analysis of large numbers of studies. Some work was also done on the contribution of various factors to outcome. It was found, for example, that treatment outcome was better when patient and therapist clarified goals for the treatment (Wilkins, 1979).

Many questions from the seventies continued into the eighties. One concerns length of treatment. Although this is a very gross measure of what takes place in treatment, there is some suggestion that each session adds to the likelihood of a good outcome only up to a point (probably around 26 sessions), and, after that, the additional value of the remainder is less clear (Howard, Kopta, Krause, & Orlinsky, 1986).

Single case studies have taken yet another new form. Detailed analysis of the language of tape-recorded session attempts to trace the psychological changes within and between sessions. This is highly labor-intensive work and a gamble for the researchers who undertake it. Another new trend is the use of manuals that instruct the psychotherapists who participate in controlled trials. This method attempts to hold constant, as much as possible, the type of active therapeutic ingredient supplied to the patients who are in the experimental group.

A Few Words for the Consumer

Before I take a closer look at how psychoanalytic ideas can play a role in a scientific view of psychotherapy, let me say a few words about the many research trends I have seen come and go in my time. The argumentative atmosphere of psychotherapy research should not frighten us away from drawing some well-warranted conclusions:

1. Treatment helps, even if we cannot prove why this is so.
2. If a patient is more intelligent, this fact tends to increase his chances of a positive treatment outcome. (Intelligence is usually a plus, so this is hardly a surprise. Besides, its effect is not a statistically strong one.)
3. In general, patients respond well to therapists who are warm, genuine, and care about patients' problems. The quality of the relationship between therapist and patient seems to be important, at least for a large class of patients.

It would be a mistake, however, to ascribe the success of psychotherapy simply to the effect of the "psychotherapeutic personality" of the therapist, as has sometimes been suggested (e.g., by Whitehorn). I believe that such a therapeutic personality is indeed helpful—like bed rest and chicken soup for an infection and fever—but to be optimally useful and effective, I would rather have the psychotherapeutic equivalent of penicillin, or even better, of a specific antibiotic typed by a culture of material taken from the patient. *Similarly, I believe that rational and scientific psychotherapy must be based on specific interventions lawfully related to a body of psychological theory.*

A few warnings should be kept in mind by the scientifically trained reader who wishes to dig into this work himself. The field is *very* uneven. Do not let the large number of poor or simple-minded studies convince you that the task is impossible.

When you read findings, look for details about the five factors mentioned in the last section (patient, situation, time, therapist, and therapeutic method). Who were the patients? How were they selected? What kinds of problems did they have? Under what conditions was therapy dispensed? Was it time limited? If so, how was this determined? What was the training of the therapist? How experienced was she or he? Did the therapist in fact embody the espoused therapeutic method? How was this fact determined?

Methods

Along with my attachment to logical positivist attitudes, my training in the psychology department at Harvard made it natural that, from my earliest days as a psychoanalyst, I wanted to ask some skeptical questions about the psychoanalytic ideas that attracted me. They seemed convincing, but I knew all too well that it was possible to fool oneself. I tried to bring a scientific attitude to my clinical work from the start, but it was not until the 1950s that I had the time and resources to organize a systematic program of research on clinical psychoanalysis.

This was no easy matter. In the early days of psychological research on psychoanalysis, there was an unfortunate tendency for concepts to be operationalized unrealistically and vaguely. Often this trend was coupled with a barely disguised hostile attitude toward clinical work on the part of the investigators. Not surprisingly, clinicians scoffed at the experimental oversimplifications and grumbled at the attitude they sensed. Understandably, they wanted to conclude that research had nothing to offer. At times, this conclusion was so ingrained that entire institutes were oblivious to the paradox of training men and women in a discipline devoted to scientific skepticism, and yet preserving their distance from the discipline of research.

Right from the start, I knew my belief in measurement put me in the minority among psychoanalysts. Most share Freud's negative feelings about quantification, believing it not only impossible but also misleading and pseudoscientific when applied to psychoanalysis. And quite frankly, when compared to the drama of psychological change, questions of measurement, prediction, falsification, and the like have seemed a bit dry to analysts.

Nevertheless, since these questions are important for anyone who views psychotherapy in a scientific light, I wanted to find a way to introduce rigorous methods that would not be so foreign to the psychoanalytic process. My tactic has been to draw on connections between scientific tools and what actually takes place in the analytic work.

I believe, for example, that the psychoanalytic distrust of quantification is a result of narrow experience. Many analysts think only of intensive scales such as the metric scale, with equal distances between stops and proportionality. Yet, since the work of my teacher S. S. Stevens, it has been recognized that one can profitably speak of nominal, ordinal, cardinal, and other scales. Not so long ago, physics too had to be satisfied with some ordinal scales, such as the relative hardness scale (e.g., talcum is softer than carborundum, but carborundum is softer than diamonds, etc.).

As discussed in Chapter One, ordinal scales can still be very usefully applied in psychological measurements and to psychoanalytic propositions. For instance, analysts may say one person is more "anal" than another, and less so than somebody else. Indeed, psychoanalysts continuously use quantitative statements without even being aware of it. They speak of patients with a strong transference or a less one, and of severe anxiety or little anxiety. Why, then, are they so reluctant to take the next step and apply numbers to these impressions, especially when the potential gain in knowledge may be significant?

Along with measurement, there is prediction. A close look at how analysts work shows that prediction takes place all the time. Every time an analyst makes an interpretation, he makes inferences by postdiction and prediction without being aware of it. (G. W. Allport used the word *postdiction* to describe a retrospective reconstruction.) In the case of an agoraphobic, for example, the analyst might say, "You are afraid of open spaces because you feel exposed. It is your way of warding off forbidden exhibitionistic impulses." Here, part of the analyst's inference is based in postdiction; he utilizes actual historical data, such as the fact that the patient grew up in a setting that forbade exhibitionism and made it very unlikely. The analyst predicts that this interpretation will have certain effects at different stages of the interactive therapeutic process—that the patient will have an anxiety dream with a theme relating to voyeurism-exhibitionism, that the interpretation of fear of exhibitionism will "roll back" this defense and evoke a need for voyeurism as primary to the need for exhibitionism. The analyst might know that the patient, as a boy, discovered that girls have no penis, a visual experience that scared him. The boy wishes to cope with this anxiety and reassure himself by exhibiting his penis. This wish is in conflict with both his ego and superego, and thus a symptom is formed.

The analytic work is thus formed of hypotheses that organize data. Indeed, I have used this thought as the basis for my method of brief psychotherapy.

Let me illustrate. In the initial interview, I want to hear all the details of the patient's complaints. When did they begin? When might they have existed before in the patient's life? I also want a detailed life history, starting at birth. What were the living conditions? Who slept where? What was the ambiance in the home? What was the ethnic, socioeconomic, and geographical setting? Who were the other family members—siblings, parents, grandparents, uncles, and aunts—and what were they like?

As I listen to the patient, I form certain hypotheses about life conditions that should have been present to produce these particular symptoms, as well as other pathology that might be expected.

Learning about the intense voyeurism of the patient, I postulate that he must have been overstimulated as a child. When I hear that the parents used to take summer vacations in a nearby sea resort, I ask for more details. It turns out that the mother and children spent a month there with the father joining the family on Friday nights. The cottage was small. It seems likely that Friday night was intercourse night, and that in the small cottage the little boy had to be aware of it. Children usually feel scared and stimulated by parental intercourse. The heavy breathing, the moaning, the movements in bed sound like aggression—aggression of the father against the mother.

I form yet another hypothesis and ask the patient for details about life during the week. I hear that this was a world without adult males, just mothers and children. In the freedom of a summer place by the sea, the ladies would talk uninhibitedly and did not think it mattered if the little boy saw them nude in the shower.

I postulate that this patient must have been overstimulated at an early age. I wonder what other symptoms this might have produced. I make the collateral inference that this man should also show some sexual problems. My first guess is that he probably suffers from what the Army used to call "piss shyness," that he cannot urinate unless he has complete privacy. I make yet another inference that he may suffer from premature ejaculation, where ejaculation is equated with urination. It turns out that I am right on both scores.

In the next session, we start the treatment process. I predict that before long the patient will relate that he also suffers from erythrophobia (a fear of blushing). Now to further the scientific process in the manner I have suggested, in the following session I would have to record a number of hypotheses, ranked in order of likelihood of occurrence. Three colleagues of mine would then watch videotapes of my sessions. Each will rank order a choice of hypotheses from 0 to 10. A high correlation between their predictions and mine would be necessary for verification of a hypothesis. On viewing the tapes, three other colleagues will formulate hypotheses. They will "judge" each hypothesis by doing their own rank ordering and formulating new hypotheses.

It is hoped that after some practice in rating, the judges will show satisfactory interrater reliability, that the predictors will show such interrater reliability for their group, and that there will also be a high correlation between predictions and judgment.

While this process might lead to the validation of some psychoanalytic hypotheses, it will prove equally valuable in examining those instances in which we find a lack of such interrater reliability and of construct validity. One such example would be if the postdictions turn out to be incorrect in terms of the actual history of the patient. Such failures will lead us to allow a longer period for trial and error, to better train the raters.

My inferences, predictions, and postdictions are the work of the treatment. At the same time, with a little effort and technical knowhow, they can be made into tools of science. In my project, my hope was to do justice to actual analytic practices, yet also introduce scientific rigor.

An Early Effort

Along with some colleagues, I have set out to introduce into the conduct of analysis the tools I have described (Bellak, 1956). After a shakedown cruise of our methodology using other patients, the sessions of two target patients in psychoanalysis were recorded for about 50 sessions each. Transcripts were typed and, because we wanted to include the sort of material that can today be captured by videotape, comments on tone of voice, body posture, and so on were added by the analyst to supplement the auditory record. A group was assembled of graduates and members of the New York Psychoanalytic Association who belonged to approximately the same academic generation. (I wanted to min-

A Form of Treatment and a Subject of Research   149

imize variability and disagreements in ratings due to differences in professional socialization.) Some made predictions; others judged the session material.

Each week transcripts were distributed. Two members tried to make predictions regarding what would happen in the next session, the next week, and in the next month. If a participant wanted to listen to the recording, he could (but this seldom occurred). Starting a week after the predictors, two judges judged what had happened in the sessions. The treating analyst also made predictions, but these were not communicated to the participants. Both groups used basically similar forms so that the predictions could be compared with the results.

As I have explained, my time at Harvard left me with a good deal of respect for quantification when it can be done intelligently, so an important goal of the project was to develop workable forms for quantifying and evaluating clinically rich material. In this study, predictors rated a number of variables, such as transference and acting out. Numbers were used (e.g., a positive transference of 2 was not very much, whereas a positive transference of 8 was quite high). The judges used an almost identical sheet.

A qualitative sheet was also included. Predictors were asked to say why they anticipated changes in a variable. On another page, they were asked to postdict the same information. Finally, on the last page, a thumbnail sketch of the week's analysis was requested; in this "freer" form, there was no need to quantify.

For 24 weeks, we met every month. Statistical findings were presented and any modifications needed were made. After the meeting, predictors and judges switched roles. Different predictors and judges were paired, varying the combinations in a systematic way. We followed this procedure first for one patient treated by another analyst, and then for another patient under my care. For this second patient, we added new hypotheses based on our findings and reformulations with the first. Naturally, since I was the treating analyst for the second patient, I could not attend the monthly meeting because I would be affected by hearing the predictions and judgments of the group. However, by this time the project was in full swing, so my absence was no problem.

We used correlation coefficients to see how well predictions fit with what the judges found. All the correlations were positive; most were moderately or strongly so. Of course, we could only include ratings when there was a high level of agreement among the judges. And, I should add, the ratings were only made on those variables rated by all the participants. (Remember, they did not have to rate each variable every time.)

A similar research study, using brief therapy as a modality for prediction and judgment, was considerably more successful. Though both research projects were shoestring operations, they were headed in the right direction and clearly demonstrated the possibility of studying the psychoanalytic process.

Despite the modest nature of our findings, I still consider this study to have been an important one. First, we showed that recording analytic sessions, if done in a tactful and responsible manner, need not interfere with the treatment process. Second, we proved that clinically rich research could be carried out in a rigorous way and that judges could agree on the basic themes running through an hour or a series of hours. Third, we showed that a *predictive* method could be used.

Even as we examined our findings, I saw many shortcomings. We needed to study both smaller and larger units—analysis usually takes years, and so predictions should aim for longer periods. Also, Rene Spitz made an important point in conversation. He said that one ought to predict the immediate response of the patient to a statement by the analyst. This kind of study should be pursued with vigor.

In less complex research, using the method of intensive design and repeated prediction and judgment, some colleagues and I were able to demonstrate the feasibility of showing changes in psychotherapy, combined with drug therapy as measured by ego function change, an approach I describe in Chapter Six (Bellak, Chassan, Gediman, & Hurvich, 1973). Ego function assessment was also used successfully in following the analytic process of a patient in supervision. This was also done by Ciompi and his associates in Bern.

Some Contemporary Examples

When my colleagues and I initiated the detailed study of transcribed recordings of treatment, we believed we had seen the future. We were right. Today, transcript studies are a staple of psychotherapy research. Their utility is enhanced by new technology. Researchers today can use word processors. In some cases, it is now possible to write programs that automatically identify and tabulate particularly interesting features of syntax or word choice. One can doubt that this type of investigation will ever take the place of line-by-line examination, yet still envy the ability to quantify at the touch of a finger.

As I have already made clear, not all psychotherapy research is psychoanalytic, but since my main interest is the overlap of psychoanalysis and research, I have chosen to illustrate some additional features of the contemporary scene (e.g., by looking briefly at the approaches taken by psychoanalysts Hartvig Dahl and Lester Luborsky). I will then discuss the psychoanalytic work of Joseph Weiss and the Mt. Zion project and several others.

When a psychoanalyst decides to study psychoanalysis or psychoanalytically oriented psychotherapy empirically, he must first answer some basic questions. Chief among them is: When I need to use technical terms to describe and explain the processes I uncover, shall I use previously existing psychoanalytic terms (e.g., *ego, displacement, transference,* etc.) or shall I start fresh with brand new terms or terms drawn from other fields such as linguistics or cognitive psychology? Even though I felt some dissatisfaction with ambiguities in existing psychoanalytic terms, I chose to carry them over into my research once they had been properly clarified (e.g., detailing the components of ego functioning). Luborsky and Dahl have used a different approach, with the former developing the useful concept of the Core Conflictual Relationship Theme, and the latter giving a special meaning to the concept of "frame," based on Marvin Minsky's (1975) use of the term in computer modeling of mental processes. (The reader who wants to learn more about these and other related research programs is referred to the volume edited by Dahl, Kächele, and Thomä [1988], which I used for my summaries.)

Luborsky's concept grew out of a concern with the measurement of transference. He had previously developed a measure of the helping alliance in treatment, and he wondered how it might fit into a more general measure of relationship patterning. As he studied transcripts of sessions, Luborsky found his attention drawn to what he called "relationship episodes" (REs), which are essentially stories the patient told regarding some interaction with another person. Again and again, he found that the key to the relationship pattern consisted of understanding three basic components, which became the components of the Core Conflictual Relationship Theme (CCRT): (1) the patient's wish, need, or intention directed toward another person in the story (labeled W); (2) the other person's response (labeled RO); and (3) the self-response of the patient (labeled RS). Over time, it has been found that these components can be reliably coded and used to investigate many aspects of the psychotherapy process.

Like Luborsky, Dahl takes as his basic data the manifest content found in transcribed sessions, which is then examined to identify repetitive structures ("frames") in the patient's material. Although the frame has a rather complex technical meaning, for our purpose we can oversimplify: Essentially, a frame is like a mental format. Most adults, for instance, have such a format for job interviews, and they organize their actions, feelings, and expectations accordingly. The interview starts with a handshake, and then continues with pleasantries, questions and answers, summary, closing, and a last handshake. Similarly, a patient might exhibit his reliance on a format in which, for instance, he expects disapproval when he seeks support. Such mental formats shape his feelings, actions, and so on.

In the CCRT, the three fundamental components are quite general. According to Dahl, frames are individualized; that is, they are patterns repeated in identical or almost identical form throughout the course of a treatment. These patterns can be used to gain information about a patient's wish-defense organization. Dahl's system requires that (1) the evidence for the existence of a frame be clearly and explicitly specified, (2) the event sequence that makes up a frame be repeated, and (3) the frame be used to make falsifiable predictions. Data are now being collected on the reliability of the identifying frame structures, and on their presence in the behavior of young children.

Joseph Weiss and the Mt. Zion Project

I suspect that if Freud could read the studies of psychotherapy that have been produced by the Mt. Zion group, he would take back some of the opinions I have quoted so far. This group's well-formulated concern with theory testing would convince him that the science had nothing to fear from the therapy. And their careful accumulation of evidence would show him that the choice between large-scale statistics and case studies was an unnecessary one. Provided sufficient control is introduced, concentrating on detailed evaluation of a small number of cases can provide persuasive evidence. Of course, I have my criticisms of Mt. Zion's work (e.g., they are a bit too trusting of process notes) but I regard it as a clear demonstration not only of the contemporary feasibility of psychotherapy research but also of the proposition that the preceding years of refinement of the field has been productive.

Starting in 1958 and relying, at first, on rather informal and uncontrolled single case studies, Joseph Weiss began to treat different psychoanalytic opinions as hypotheses to be tested. For example, he wondered if a patient exercised some unconscious control over the emerging consciousness of mental material that had been repressed. Or was this coming into consciousness an uncontrolled breakthrough of material? He also wondered about the best way to understand these moments, familiar to any therapist, when a patient makes some sort of demand on him. Was this the patient's way of testing the therapist—seeing if he would surrender neutrality and respond to the demand—or was it an attempt to gratify an unconscious impulse? Early on, these alternatives were empirically evaluated by inspecting process notes. Starting in 1964, Harold Sampson joined forces with Weiss in the development of complex, sophisticated methods that the Mt. Zion research group has used to test these and other hypotheses that have grown from their work.

The two early questions Weiss asked have an element in common. He considered two pairs of alternatives. In each pair, one alternative pictures the unconscious mind functioning in a more or less automatic fashion. Weiss and Sampson say this picture comes from early Freud. In the *Interpretation of Dreams* (1900), Freud played down the individual's ability to exert even minimal control over any aspect of unconscious functioning. Impulses seek gratification. Defenses stand in their way. Forces clash. Stronger forces overcome weak ones. Equal forces check one another. Occasionally, tangential forces result in compromises in which each force partly achieves its aim. Nothing, or almost nothing, that happens in the unconscious takes account of the patient's thoughts, beliefs, or assessment of reality. For obvious reasons, Weiss and Sampson chose to call this the "hypothesis of automatic functioning."

As they see the matter, however, Freud later developed an alternative view. As early as in *Inhibitions, Symptoms, and Anxiety* (1926a), Freud suggested a person may hold on to his psychopathology in obedience to certain beliefs. And, in *An Outline of Psychoanalysis* (1940), Freud stated (without elaborating) his belief that a person may be able to regulate unconsciously his behavior, basing his actions on thoughts, beliefs, and assessments of reality. In this unconscious regulation, the "ego is governed by considerations of safety" (Freud, 1940, p. 199). This is referred to as the "hypothesis of higher mental functioning."

Weiss and Sampson believe—correctly, in my opinion—that most analysts assume the existence of both automatic and higher mental functioning in unconscious processes. However, they also believe—and here I am not sure they are correct—that the automatic functioning hypothesis is "more prominent in current psychoanalytic literature [and] exerts the greater influence on present-day clinical thinking" (1986, p. 23). Predecessors to this division of ideas are freely acknowledged, such as my analyst Ernst Kris's frequently iterated point that the ego may control aspects of the unconscious (in the regression it undertakes in artistic fantasy, or in the coming into consciousness of warded-off memories, brought forth to help it attain mastery over the unconscious).

The Mt. Zion group believes the role of higher mental functions has been wrongly neglected. But, unlike many analysts who today reject the picture of the mind as an automatic interplay of forces, Weiss and Sampson are not making a *philosophical* objection to the hypothesis of automatic functioning; the unconscious might very well function in that way. The only method of choosing between this hypothesis and the hypothesis of higher mental functioning is an empirical test.

Empirical consequences were deduced from two hypotheses. For example, the researchers asked: If a patient presents a neurotic need to the analyst and the analyst responds neutrally instead of gratifying that need, what will be the result? The automatic functioning hypothesis says that the failure to gratify the impulses behind these needs will lead to frustration, tension, and conflict. The higher mental functioning hypothesis, as amended by the assumption that the patient comes into treatment to test unconscious pathogenic beliefs, says that there will be circumstances when the patient will be greatly relieved to find that the need was not gratified.

Many efforts have been made to guard against bias.

The Mt. Zion group used process notes and summaries, and transcribed analytic sessions of a tape recorded analysis by an analyst in another city, one unfamiliar with their issues who was pretty much in accordance with the automatic functioning hypothesis. They used 19 different measures of the patient's behavior and 5 of the analyst's behavior. Each measure was scored or rated by at least two independent judges; efforts were made to limit the information available to the absolute minimum needed for coding, rating, or measuring the instance. For example, if a judge was rating assertiveness, he had no idea whether material came from an earlier or later session. And, if the same response by the patient was to be rated on several different measures, a separate group of judges rated each measure, so that they would not be influenced by the rating they gave it on a previous measure.

The many studies reported in Weiss and Sampson (1986) were based on the analysis of a woman they called Mrs. C. She came into treatment for sexual problems, an inability to have orgasms during intercourse. As they came to see the matter, her behavior was controlled by an unconscious pathogenic belief that her well-being deprived her family and made them envious. She also unconsciously believed that her independence harmed them. She expressed her loyalty to her parents by identifying with their worst traits.

According to their formulation, Mrs. C. came into treatment with an unconscious plan to change her pathogenic beliefs by testing them with the analyst. For example, she displayed her abilities and independence to see if this would harm the analyst or cause him to disapprove. During the first 100 sessions, Mrs. C.'s analyst said little, though he drew her attention to her difficulties in free associating and her avoidance of certain topics. Despite his inactivity, all the evidence pointed to progress. Experienced analysts, unfamiliar with Mt. Zion's hypotheses, said Mrs. C. improved. She became more relaxed, happier, less driven, and was able to have orgasm during intercourse. Why?

In the various studies, it was found that, with little or

no interpretive help, she became aware of repressed material and aware that her fears of asserting herself were irrational. Raters agreed that she worked in accordance with the unconscious plan formulated by the research project. And, during the termination phase, she formulated a plan to test her pathogenic beliefs that leaving treatment was bad and readily agreed with interpretations in accord with this plan.

Useful as the work of Sampson and Weiss is, they sometimes used their notes as primary data. That always leaves open what they might have missed, including tone of voice and facial expressions. Certainly audiotaping throughout (as I used in my study, "An Experimental Study of the Psychoanalytic Process") or, even better, videotaping would have been much more desirable. Altogether, I don't find their demonstration of cause and effect in changes of the psychoanalytic process entirely convincing. I consider the method used in my study mentioned above much tighter—that of repeated prediction and judgment.

The basic scientific requirement that operations relating to scientific inference be publicly demonstrable and repeatable can now be fulfilled by the advent of videotape technology. Let us suppose that the American Psychoanalytic Association or the National Institute of Mental Health sponsors a program of videotaped recordings of 100 analysis patients being treated for agoraphobia. It would then be possible to study these life histories, symptom formations, and personalities for common denominators and variations. These data would permit some basic verification, rejection, or modification of existing hypotheses.

Hope for the Future

One of the most promising developments in recent years is a landmark meeting dedicated solely to controlled experimental research in psychoanalysis. On April 5 and 6 of 1991, a section of the International Psychoanalytic Association (IPA) met at the University of London Hospital Center. About 200 people took part in the conference. It was an especially joyous experience for me to attend, since I had lobbied for IPA-sponsored research for decades (e.g., in a 1977 letter to Serge Lebovici, who later published it in his presidential newsletter). Also, in 1976, I corresponded with Robert Wallerstein, later president of the American Psychoanalytic Association (APA), concerning their sponsorship of controlled research. Still, it took more organizational acumen than I had to translate these ideas into fact. Both Wallerstein and Joseph Sandler, who succeeded Wallerstein as President of the IPA, worked to arrange for this conference in London—a task that required much diplomacy, since in both organizations there is still a strong conservative trend that considers controlled research antithetical to psychoanalysis. Consider, for instance, that an entire issue of the *Psychoanalytic Quarterly* (volume LIX, no. 4, 1990) was dedicated to a discussion of the psychoanalytic process—with only one brief reference to experimental studies by Allan Compton and a bibliographic reference by Arlow and Brenner to my own research in 1956. There was no response to a critical letter of mine from editors or contributors, except by Compton and Brenner.

As of this writing, it will still take considerable work and fortitude to obtain organizational approval from the section on research in the IPA. Even further away from realization is my earlier suggestion that the IPA and APA should become the recipients and disbursers of grants for the support of research as well as the initiator of research projects.

Such scenarios are indeed possible: In 1963, I testified before the U.S. Congress that it was vital to establish a Center for Schizophrenia Research at NIMH. This action stemmed from my growing concern that research in schizophrenia suffered from a lack of both communication and centralization. Such a center, I believed, should publish relevant studies very promptly and should sponsor research out of its own budget; it should also engage in research where it felt a deficiency and integrate its findings with other research work. Since that time, the center has indeed played a central role in schizophrenia research, albeit without sufficient financial support for seed money. I feel strongly that a similar organizational approach will prove useful in the field of psychoanalysis.

Robert Wallerstein has also formulated a new plan: a collaborative, multisite program of psychoanalytic therapy research. In the proposed project, a group of 15 people would collaborate in a study of the psychoanalytic process based on microscopic scrutiny of audio-recorded psychoanalytic hours, using instruments that they themselves had developed. They would then apply these methods and measurements to the study of identical sessions drawn from a pool of audio-recorded psychoanalyses. Admittedly, there will be tremendous obstacles to overcome, such as facilitating the remarkably complex (but necessary) safeguarding of both patient and analyst identities. However, the program is extremely ambitious and worthwhile, and should be an excellent candidate for foundation support.

Some of the reports from the London conference indicated real progress along the lines of systematic research. For instance, Thomä and Kächele discussed their ongoing work in Ulm (see below), which has been supported by the Volkswagen Foundation and the German government. Otto Kernberg, who was involved in the Menninger project of research in psychotherapy, together with many others still active in psychoanalytic research, has continued his work of observing the clinical process of the psychoanalysis of a borderline patient. Howard Shevrin spoke in London (and also a few weeks later at the New York Psychoanalytic Institute) about his studies of the convergence of conscious symptoms and unconscious words related to the patient's conscious experience (e.g., of a phobia), and the hypothesized underlying conflict. He was able to show that patterns of brain frequencies differentiate between conscious symptom experience and unconscious conflict. One must hope that such studies of cognition and neurophysiological processes, as well as the controlled studies of transference, will eventually inform clinical psychoanalytic practice, much as basic scientific research informs medical practices.

My personal preference is, in fact, for studies that are more closely related to clinical problems. I have mentioned the necessity of having a tape library of patients with various ailments in order to establish why some develop an obsessive-compulsive neurosis and others a phobia. The more we learn about specifics, the more effective our therapy should be, and the more valuable our contribution to prevention will be.

At the conference in London, it also became apparent that there is an abundance of researchers in psychoanalysis who are mostly concerned with studying the psychoanalytic process rather than its outcome. There are many definitions for the psychoanalytic process, also discussed in *Psychoanalytic Quarterly*. For me, a simple definition suffices: The psychoanalytic process consists of an interaction between patient and psychoanalyst, predicated on psychoanalytic hypotheses, with an eventual goal of producing beneficial changes in the patient.

Many of these researchers have developed methods of their own to measure these changes; a surprisingly large number are concerned with cognitive and grammatical data, often quite observation-distant. Almost all of these researchers work in the United States. A major exception to both of these "rules" is the research center in Ulm (mentioned above) under the direction of H. Thomä and Horst Kächele. Over a period of more than a decade, they have accumulated what they call the "Ulm text bank." They have recorded a very large number of analyses, often lasting for years. Not only have they studied this record themselves but they have also made it available to any number of workers. They also exchange data with the research centers directed by Marti Horowitz in San Francisco and Hartvig Dahl in New York, both of whom have primarily studied shorter (five-minute) sections of patients' communications. Both the Ulm group and Horowitz have also fulfilled a very important scientific necessity: By studying each others' patients as well as their own, they tested interrater reliability.

The Dahl, Thomä, and Kächele volume, *Psychoanalytic Process Research Strategies* (1988), gives an overview of much that is going on in the field, discussing single case study methods, time-series analyses of psychoanalytic treatment processes in a single case, and problems in audio recording psychoanalytic sessions. General problems of methodology in clinical psychoanalytic research are also examined in *Problems of Metascience and Methodology in Clinical Psychoanalytic Research* (1975), and in *Psyche: Zeitschrift für Psychoanalyse und ihr Anwendungen, Herausgegeben von Alexander Mitscherlich* (1976).

Elsewhere there is related work by Horowitz on conscious and unconscious mental processes, supported by the John D. and Catherine T. MacArthur Foundation. In his introduction to *Program on Conscious and Unconscious Processes* (1991), Horowitz states,

> *The aim of this program is to develop a scientific understanding of how unconscious organizing processes affect thought and produce phenomena such as repetitive irrational choices, intrusive ideas and emotions, recurring erroneous conceptions of others, distorted self-appraisals, and forgetting or avoidance of important life events or tasks. Knowledge from the study of these phenomena would be used to develop further theories about conscious representations and unconscious formative processes, and to suggest new ways in which neurotic psychopathology might be treated or prevented.*

One way in which I personally have tried to understand this body of work is to remind myself that *unconscious*—used as an adjective—has many meanings, as I have discussed elsewhere (Spence, 1967), and that some unconscious structures were formerly conscious. My favorite hypothesis about the process by which they become unconscious is predicated on the teachings of *Gestalt* psychology—that an experience is modified by future experiences so that figure is made into ground or into other figures. The earlier experience is thus rendered "unconscious" (i.e., not accessible under ordinary circumstances). As discussed in Chapter Three, this sum total of past apperceptions, or apperceptive mass (Murray, 1943), has, in turn, a structuring effect on daily experience, and is to a certain extent similar to what Horowitz, Dahl, and others refer to as *thema*. The latter is a term that Henry A. Murray used similarly in his *Explorations in Personality: A Clinical and Experimental Study of Fifty Men of College Age* (1938): "A *thema* may be defined as the dynamical structure of a simple episode, a single creature-environment interaction" (p. 42). Then, an excursion into physiology: "It may prove convenient to refer to the mutually dependent processes that constitute dominant configurations in the brain as *regnant* processes; and, further, to designate the totality of such processes occurring during a single moment (a unitary temporal segment of brain processes) as a *regnancy*" (p. 45).

For me, the apperceptive mass (Bellak, 1954) *is what psychoanalysis tries to "analyze" through the method of free association; that is, making previous gestalten conscious again in order to restructure them into less maladaptive configurations.*

Gestalt psychology not only provides the best theoretical framework for the understanding of dreams (i.e., a *gestalt* that consists of kaleidoscopic combinations of perceptions from different times in a dreamer's life) but it is also especially helpful in understanding hypnagogic and hypnopompic phenomena. In these processes one can actually perceive a combination of present and past apperceptions (e.g., the perception of the actual process of falling asleep or waking up). *Gestalt* psychology can also illuminate one's comprehension of hallucinations and delusions. Hallucinations in particular are characterized by a weakening of the boundaries of figure and ground. Most hallucinations start as accurate perceptions but turn into illusions. Then, with further weakening of the figure-ground definition, illusions—which are often merely poor attempts at adaptation—turn into full-fledged hallucinations.

It is, in short, regrettable that *Gestalt* psychology and the work of Murray are not better known, especially among medical analysts. The application of this knowledge to psychoses offers a wealth of clinically important material that remains primarily untapped.

Conclusion: The Future

Having discussed psychotherapy research, what can be said about its future?

Thus far, technology has played an important role. With each new recording device, new types of data have been made available. Today, frame-by-frame analyses can be made of videotaped facial expressions, gestures, and the like. Muscle patterns in the face can be reliably detected and coded to indicate emotions. Tone of voice can be quantified. Sophisticated psycholinguistic analysis of word choice can be made. And, most importantly, huge quantities of data over extended period of time can be aggregated. Using newly powerful statistical techniques that correct for chance correlations and observation of fluctuations and trends that would likely be invisible to even the most discerning clinical eye, statistical tests can be conducted that Freud never dreamed possible.

New developments in electronic technology now appear much faster than researchers can assimilate. We can expect this trend to continue in the foreseeable future. We will be limited only by the "mind-forged manacles" we impose on ourselves: lack of imagination, outworn ideologies, and sentimental attitudes.

I must express both a fear and a hope regarding this new psychotherapy research. My fear is that it will fail to flourish just as it is coming into its own because the current, quite biologically oriented *Zeitgeist* in psychiatry may wrongly equate the biological with the scientific. As I have made clear throughout this book, science is not to be identified with a specific subject matter but with a skeptical attitude of mind and with a methodology. A biological psychiatrist who is interested in biological findings because he finds them scientifically convincing is no threat to psychotherapy research, because he will simply demand evidence—which is as it should be. But a biological psychiatrist whose preference for brain-based findings is an article of faith has given up the scientific spirit.

Only the future will determine whether this new psychotherapy research will flourish, but my hope is that it may be assisted by an unlikely source. Sources of third-party payments are more interested in money than they are in science, biology, or psychotherapy. We can expect them to care about evidence of effectiveness, not about types of intervention. If this is the case—that is, if psychotherapy can be shown to be cost effective—then research on the processes involved in it can expect to get a healthy cure for the declining revenues of the mental health sector of the economy.

Epilogue

What is the future of psychoanalysis? This question is often the topic of heated discussions. The *Psychoanalytic Quarterly* devoted a series of lead articles to precisely that topic in 1990. Yet, the basic distinction needed to answer that question reasonably is usually made neither in meetings nor in the *Quarterly*—and that is the distinction between psychoanalysis as a form of therapy and psychoanalysis as a theory of personality.

I am most uncertain about the future of psychoanalysis as a form of treatment. The temper of our time speaks against its flowering. We live in a culture of great mobility. The chances of someone staying in one place for an average of four years are relatively small. This is especially true during one's younger years of climbing up the corporate ladder. The ability to afford the time and money for four or five times a week on the couch is getting slimmer. The financial burden has always been a great one for both patient and analyst. In the case of the analyst, remember that he must attempt to fashion a living out of a very few patients, since each one is seen for 50 minutes, and one can see at most only 8 or 9 patients a day. Because of that limitation, the cost to the individual patient is quite high, if the psychoanalyst is to have a living consonant with that of other clinicians. It is the latter fact that makes the general public feel that all psychoanalysts much be rich when, in fact, repeated surveys have shown them to be at the bottom of the income level for medical specialties. The situation for nonmedical therapists is only slightly better compared to that of their peers. In either case, third-party payers are rarely willing to cover more than a fraction of the cost of psychoanalysis. Thus, any number of therapeutic approaches are competing successfully with psychoanalysts for the therapy dollar.

One can only hope that analysis in its classical form will survive as training for psychiatrists and other mental health professionals; that it will serve as a broad base for their understanding of personality and character, and to utilize the interpretation of art for derivative forms of psychotherapy.

For psychoanalysis as a theory of personality, the situation is quite different. From its shaky beginnings about a century ago (*The Interpretation of Dreams* was published in 1900) Freud's basic theory of personality basically stands alone, above all other theories and psychotherapies built upon it. Classical Freudian psychoanalytic theory stands on the firm foundation of causality, on the basic principles of learning, of perception, and of all the other facets I have mentioned previously.

I have tried to show that psychoanalysis as a theory of personality is grounded in the basic principles of causality, not the complex causality of quantum mechanics or of abstruse philosophy, but rather the down-to-earth causality that we rely upon when we are driving a car or cooking a meal. Psychoanalysis as a personality theory is, essentially, homely.

Predicated on this simple foundation, the psychoanalytic theory of personality then builds a very complex house of interlocking hypotheses. It proposes to undo the effects of the past by formulating another group of hypotheses including postdiction and prediction. Treatment, therefore, is a lawful form of unlearning and relearning, employing a variety of means—particularly insight—to change internalized *Gestalten,* to produce different, more adaptive coping.

I have pointed out that most medical psychoanalysts have usually not been trained in concept formation or methodology. They are barely aware that they have regularly employed a variety of learning theories in order to correct earlier, often maladaptive, behavior.

As I have also attempted to demonstrate, psychoanalysts have not been precise in their understanding of their learning hypotheses, nor have they clearly stated the nature and interaction of these hypotheses. I refer the reader back to the academic learning concept of the laws of primacy and frequency, and the conditioning concepts involved.

Because the psychoanalytic theory of personality has not had the benefit of good conceptualization, therapeutic learning and unlearning have not been clearly stated or maximized, or optimized in terms of time and effectiveness. There must be instances in which one form of unlearning and relearning is actually better than another. For example, learning from the transference experience may sometimes be superior to learning by insight, and vice versa.

I have also pointed out that the psychoanalytic theory of personality involves a theory of motivation, a theory of development, and other theories; yet none of these have been sufficiently examined by controlled experiments. Most of these theories have not been investigated, demonstrated, disproved, or modified at all. I believe that most of them can be so studied, and have tried to investigate some of them myself.

I have mentioned that psychoanalysis as a form of therapy may receive aid from various third-party payers. If insurance companies want to know whether psychoanalysis or psychotherapy really works before paying for it, money and energy must be made available to study the effect of such treatments in controlled, experimental ways. While this is happening to a certain extent—and is even supported for the first time by the National Institute of Mental Health—these efforts are still mostly of the primitive kind (i.e., outcome studies). It will take process studies of videotaped analyses and investigation of the minutest parts of psychoanalytic theory to prove or disprove the validity of this process.

Meanwhile, much of the discussion of the value of psychoanalysis as a form of treatment remains downright fatuous. Take, for instance, the question of superiority of behavior therapy or cognitive therapy over classical psychoanalysis, or any number of other forms of psychotherapies.

Classical psychoanalytic therapy is predicated upon the complex foundations of classical theory of personality. Thus, it allows prediction and postdiction, and also profits from the complex interaction of the therapy with motivational and developmental theories. As such, psychoanalytic theory and therapy attempt to understand and change the patient by examining not only manifest behavior but also dreams, delusions, hallucinations, and so on.

What is the theory of personality involved in cognitive therapy? How does cognitive therapy or behavioral psychology and therapy explain dreams or hallucinations?

Without belaboring the point, classical psychoanalytic therapy is superior in principle because it is based upon the rational—if not experimentally verified—theory of psychoanalytic theory, with all its complex causal connections.

This by no means implies, however, that psychoanalysis as treatment or psychoanalytic psychotherapy derived from classical analysis is always the preferred method of treatment. I myself both use and teach brief psychotherapy, because that is either all that is indicated or all that can be provided. Still, all of my brief therapy is based on classical hypotheses; that is the main reason, I believe, why it has been successful.

Also, a primarily insightful therapy may be neither indicated, possible, nor desirable. There are many instances where cognitive therapy may be the preferred method; the patient may require an awareness that the glass is not only half empty but also half full. The strategies of cognitive therapy may be very helpful in treating a patient's anxieties and depressions by giving him a different outlook, a new way of seeing himself. Still, cognitive therapy can draw on no complex theory of personality to explain the broad spectrum of human behavior.

Similarly, behavior therapy may be the most effective treatment of some severe phobias, but its principles of learning theories are primitive and severely limited.

Psychoanalytic personality theory needs to be supported and studied because it is a mother lode for applied psychoanalysis as therapy, for an understanding of psychosomatic medicine, art, and human behavior in general. In order for its optimum continuation, however, psychoanalysts should be trained in methodology and statistics, not in internecine warfare and politics.

As a form of treatment, psychoanalysis is subject to all the historical forces that are shaping our world. We don't even know if we will be able to preserve the ozone layer, so how can we predict whether technology—and the tremendous mobility of our society and its economy—will permit a person to lie on a couch for an hour, four times a week, and slowly learn, unlearn, and relearn better coping mechanisms?

Will classical psychoanalytic theory of personality survive? It will, as long as causality remains a meaningful concept; despite the limitations of only one lifetime of experience, and the uncertainty of the future and, undoubtedly, a great deal of personal bias in its defense—I am entirely certain that it will.

Bibliography

Allport, G. (1937). *Personality: A psychological interpretation.* New York: Holt.

Arlow, J., & Brenner, C. (1964). *Psychoanalytic concepts and the structural theory.* New York: International Universities Press.

Bartley, W. (1973). *Wittgenstein.* LaSalle, IL.: Open Court.

Bellak, L. (1944). The concept of projection: And experimental investigation and study of the concept. *Psychiatry, 7,* 353–370.

———. (1950). Projection and the TAT. In L. Crafts, T. Schneirla, et al. (Eds.), *Recent experiments in psychology* (rev. ed.). New York: McGraw-Hill.

———. (1954). *The Thematic Apperception Test and Children's Apperception Test in clinical use* (2nd ed.). New York: Grune & Stratton.

———. (1956). An experimental exploration of the psychoanalytic process: Exemplification of a method. *Psychoanalytic Quarterly, 25,* 385–413.

———. (1959a). Introduction: The frame of reference of the monograph. In *Conceptual and methodological problems in psychoanalysis.* Special Issue of *Annals of the New York Academy of Science, 76,* 973–975.

———. (1959b). The unconscious. In *Conceptual and methodological problems in psychoanalysis.* Special Issue of *Annals of the New York Academy of Science, 76,* 1066–1081.

———. (1961). Free association: Conceptual and clinical

aspects. *International Journal of Psychoanalysis, 42,* 9–20.

———. (forthcoming). *The TAT, CAT, and SAT in clinical use* (5th ed.). Boston: Allyn and Bacon.

Bellak, L., Chassan, J., Gediman, H., & Hurvich, J. (1973). Ego function assessment of analytic psychotherapy combined with drug therapy. *Journal of Nervous and Mental Disease, 157,* 465–469.

Bellak, L., & Ekstein, R. (1946). The extension of some basic scientific laws to psychoanalysis and to psychology. *Psychoanalytic Review, 33,* 306–311.

Bellak, L., & Goldsmith, L. (1984). *The broad scope of ego function assessment.* New York: Wiley. See also: Spence, D. (Ed.) (1967). *The broad scope of psychoanalysis: The selected papers of Leopold Bellak.* New York: Grune & Stratton.

Bellak, L., Hurvich, M., & Gediman, H. (1973). *Ego functions in schizophrenics, neurotics, and normals: A systematic study of conceptual, diagnostic and therapeutic aspects.* New York: Wiley.

Bergin, A. (1963). The effects of psychotherapy: Negative results revisited. *Journal of Consulting Psychology, 10,* 244–250.

Bernfeld, S. (1925/1973). *Sisyphus.* Berkeley: University of California Press.

Bowlby, J. (1951). Maternal care and mental health. *Bulletin of the World Health Organization, 3,* 355–534.

———. (1969). *Attachment and loss: I. Attachment.* London: Hogarth Press.

———. (1973). *Attachment and loss: II. Separation: Anxiety and anger.* London: Hogarth Press.

———. (1980). *Attachment and loss: III. Sadness and depression.* London: Hogarth Press.

———, Figlio, G., & Young, R. (1986). An interview with John Bowlby on the origins and reception of his work. *Free Association,* 36–64.

Breuer, J., & Freud, S. (1895). Studies on hysteria. In J. Strachey (Ed.), *The standard edition of the complete psychological works of Sigmund Freud, Vol. II.* London: Hogarth.

Cannon, W. (1927). The James-Lange theory of emotions: A critical re-examination and an alternative theory. *American Journal of Psychology, 39,* 106–124.
Clark, R. (1980). *Freud: The man and the cause.* New York: Random House.
Dahl, H., Kächele, H., & Thomä, H. (1988). *Psychoanalytic process research strategies.* New York: Springer-Verlag.
Drury, M. (1984). Conversations with Wittgenstein. In R. Rhees (Ed.), *Recollections of Wittgenstein.* New York: Oxford University Press.
Eagle, M. (1987). *Recent developments in psychoanalysis: A critical evaluation.* Cambridge, MA: Harvard University Press.
Erickson, E. (1950). *Childhood and society.* New York: Norton.
Eysenck, H. (1952). The effects of psychotherapy: An evaluation. *Journal of Consulting Psychology, 16,* 319–324.
———. (1960). *Behavior therapy and the neuroses.* London: Pergamon Press.
———. (1985). Psychotherapy effects: Real or imaginary. *American Psychologist, 40,* 239–240.
Fisher, S., & Greenberg, R. (1977). *The scientific credibility of Freud's theories and therapy.* New York: Basic Books.
Flew, A. (1949). Psycho-analytic explanation. *Analysis, 10,* 8–15.
———. (1956). Motives and the unconscious. In H. Feigl & M. Scriven (Eds.). *Minnesota studies in philosophy of science* (vol I.). Minneapolis: University of Minnesota Press.
Frank, P. (1959). Psychoanalysis and logical positivism. In S. Hook (Ed.), *Psychoanalysis, scientific method, and philosophy.* New York: NYU Press.
Freidlander, B. (1970). Receptive language development in infancy. *Merrill-Palmer Quarterly, 16,* 7–51.
Freud, S. (1895). Project for a scientific psychology. In J. Strachey (Ed.), *The complete psychological works of Sigmund Freud, vol. I* (pp. 281–387). London: Hogarth.

---. (1900). Interpretation of dreams. In J. Strachey (Ed.), *The complete psychological works of Sigmund Freud, vol. 4–5* (pp. 1–622). London: Hogarth.

---. (1905). Three essays on a theory of sexuality. In J. Strachey (Ed.), *The complete psychological works of Sigmund Freud, vol. 7* (pp. 1–243). London: Hogarth.

---. (1909). Analysis of a phobia in a five-year-old boy. In J. Strachey (Ed.), *The complete psychological works of Sigmund Freud, vol. 10* (pp. 1–150). London: Hogarth.

---. (1913). Totem and taboo. In J. Strachey (Ed.), *The complete psychological works of Sigmund Freud, vol. 13* (pp. 1–162). London: Hogarth.

---. (1920). Beyond the pleasure principle. In J. Strachey (Ed.), *The complete psychological works of Sigmund Freud, vol. 18* (pp. 1–66). London: Hogarth.

---. (1923). The ego and the id. In J. Strachey (Ed.), *The complete psychological works of Sigmund Freud, vol. 19* (pp. 1–66). London: Hogarth.

---. (1926a). Inhibitions, symptoms, and anxiety. In J. Strachey (Ed.), *The complete psychological works of Sigmund Freud, vol. 20* (pp. 75–176). London: Hogarth.

---. (1926b). The question of lay analysis. In J. Strachey (Ed.), *The complete psychological works of Sigmund Freud, vol. 20* (pp. 177–258). London: Hogarth.

---. (1927). *Einführung in die Technik der Kinderanalyse*. Leipzig: Internationaler Psychoanalytischer Verlag.

---. (1933). New introductory lectures. In J. Strachey (Ed.), *The complete psychological works of Sigmund Freud, vol. 22* (pp. 1–182). London: Hogarth.

---. (1936). *The ego and the mechanisms of defense*. New York: International Universities Press.

---. (1940). An outline of psychoanalysis. In J. Strachey (Ed.), *The complete psychological works of Sigmund Freud, vol. 23* (pp. 139–208). London: Hogarth.

Gadamer, H. G. (1976). *Philosophical hermeneutics* (D. E. Longe, Trans. & Ed.). Berkeley: University of California Press.

Gay, P. (1988). *Freud: A life for our time.* New York: Norton.
Greenberg, J., & Mitchell, S. (1983). *Object relations in psychoanalytic theory.* Cambridge, MA: Harvard University Press.
Greenspan, S. (1981). *Clinical infant reports: No. 1, Psychopathology and adaption in infancy in early childhood.* New York: International Universities Press.
Groddeck, G. (1923). *Das buch vom es.* Vienna: International Psychoanalytischen Verlag.
Grosskurth, P. (1986). *Melanie Klein: Her world and her work.* New York: Alfred Knopf.
Grünbaum, A. (1984). *The foundations of psychoanalysis: A philosophical critique.* Berkeley: University of California Press.
Habermas, J. (1971). *Knowledge and human interests* (J. J. Schapiro, Trans.) Boston: Beacon Press.
Harlow, H. (1971). *Learning to love.* San Francisco: Albion.
Hartmann, H. (1950). Comments on the psychoanalytic theory of the ego. In *Essays on ego psychology, 1964.* New York: International Universities Press.
Heinicke, C. (1956). Some effects of separating two-year-old children from their parents: A comparative study. *Human Relations, 9,* 105–176.
———, & Westheimer, I. (1966). *Brief separations.* New York: International Universities Press.
Hersen, M., Michelson, L., & Bellack, A. (1984). *Issues in psychotherapy research.* New York: Plenum press.
Hook, S. (1959). *Psychoanalysis, scientific method, and philosophy.* New York: NYU Press.
Horowitz, M. (1991). *Program on conscious and unconscious processes.* Unbound program flyer.
Howard, K., Kopta, S., Krause, M., & Orlinsky, D. (1986). The dose-effect relationship in psychotherapy. *American Psychologist, 41,* 159–164.
Jacoby, R. (1986). *The repression of psychoanalysis.* New York: Basic Books.
Klein, G. S. (1976). *Psychoanalytic theory.* New York: International Universities Press.
Klein, M. (1964). *Contributions to psychoanalysis, 1921–1945.* New York: McGraw-Hill.

Langer, W. & Gifford, S. (1978). An American analyst in Vienna during the Anschluss, 1936–1938. *Journal of the History of the Behavioral Sciences, 14.*

Levine, R., Chein, I., & Murphy, G. (1943). The relationship of the intensity of a need to the amount of perceptual distortion: A preliminary report. *Journal of Psychology, 13,* 283–293.

Lorenz, K. (1970). *Studies in animal and human behavior* (R. Martin, Trans.). London: Methuen.

MacFarlane, J. (1975). Olfaction in the development of social preferences in the human neonate. In M. Hofer (Ed.), *Parent-infant interaction.* Amsterdam: Elsevier.

MacIntyre, A. (1958). *The unconscious.* London: Routledge and Kegan Paul.

———. (1967). Psychoanalysis. In Paul Edward (Ed.), *Encyclopedia of Philosophy.* New York: Macmillan.

Mahler, M., Pine, F., & Bergman, A. (1975). *The psychological birth of the human infant.* New York: Basic Books.

Matarazzo, J. (1971). Research on the teaching and learning of psychotherapeutic skills. In A. Bergin & S. Garfield (Eds.), *Handbook of psychotherapy and behavior change: An empirical analysis.* New York: Wiley.

Minsky, M. (1975). A framework for representing knowledge. In P. Winston (Ed.), *The psychology of computer vision* (pp. 211–277). New York: McGraw-Hill.

Murray, H. (1938). *Explorations of personality: A clinical and experimental study of fifty men of college age.* New York: Oxford University Press.

———. (1943). *Thematic Apperception Test.* Cambridge, MA: Harvard University Press.

Peterfreund, E. (1978). Some critical comments on psychoanalytic conceptualizations of infancy. *International Journal of Psychoanalysis, 59,* 427–441.

Peters, R. (1958). *The concept of motivation.* New York: Humanities Press.

Popper, K. (1962). *Conjectures and refutations.* New York: Basic Books.

———. (1974). *Unended quest.* LaSalle, IL: Open Court.

Rapaport, D. (1957). Cognitive structures. In J. Bruner et

al. (Eds.), *Contemporary approaches to cognition* (pp. 157–200). Cambridge, MA: Harvard University Press.

Ricoeur, P. (1970). *Freud and philosophy*. New Haven, CT: Yale University Press.

Rogers, C. (1958). The necessary and sufficient conditions of therapeutic personality change. *Journal of Consulting Psychology, 21*, 95–103.

Sander, L. (1964). Adaptive relationships in early mother-child interaction. *Journal of the American Academy of Child Psychiatry, 3*, 231–264.

Schaefer, R. (1976). *A new language for psychoanalysis*. New Haven, CT: Yale University Press.

———. (1978). *Language and insight*. New Haven, CT: Yale University Press.

———. (1980). Narration in the psychoanalytic dialogue. In W. J. T. Mitchell (Ed.), *On narrative* (pp. 25–49). Chicago: University of Chicago Press.

———. (1981). *Narrative actions in psychoanalysis*. Worcester, MA: Clark University.

———. (1983). *The analytic attitude*. New York: Basic Books.

Sears, R. (1936). Experimental studies of projection: I. Attribution of traits. *Journal of Social Psychology, 7*, 151–163.

Sechehaye, M. (1955). *A symbolic realization: A new method of psychotherapy applied to a case of schizophrenia*. New York: International Universities Press.

Seebohm, T. (1977a). The problem of hermeneutics in recent Anglo-American literature: Part I. *Philosophy and Rhetoric, 10*(3), 180–198.

———. (1977b). The problem of hermeneutics in recent Anglo-American literature: Part II. *Philosophy and Rhetoric, 10*(4), 263–275.

Shapiro, D. A., & Shapiro, D. (1982). Meta-analysis of comparative therapy outcome studies: A replication and refinement. *Psychological Bulletin, 92*, 581–604.

Sheldon, W. (1954). *Atlas of men: A guide for somatotyping the adult male at all ages*. New York: Harper and Row.

Smith, M., Glass, G., & Miller, T. (1980). *The benefits of psychotherapy*. Baltimore, MD: Johns Hopkins University Press.

Spence, D. (Ed.) (1967). *The broad scope of psychoanalysis: The selected papers of Leopold Bellak*. New York: Grune & Stratton.

———. (1981). Toward a theory of dream interpretation. *Psychoanalysis and Contemporary Thought, 4*, 383–405.

———. (1982). *Narrative truth and historical truth*. New York: Norton.

———. (1983). Narrative persuasion. *Psychoanalysis and Contemporary Thought, 6*(3), 457–481.

———. (1986). When interpretation masquerades as explanation. *Journal of the American Psychoanalytic Association, 34*(1), 3–22.

Spitz, R. (1957). *No and yes: On the genesis of human communication*. New York: International Universities Press.

Stern, D. (1985). *The interpersonal world of the infant: A view from psychoanalysis and developmental psychology*. New York: Basic Books.

Thomä, H. & Kächele, H. (1988). Psychoanalytic process research strategies. Berlin: Springer Verlag.

———. (1975). Problems of metascience and methodology in clinical psychoanalytic research. New York: International Universities Press.

———. (1976). Psyche: Zeitschrift für Psychoanalyse und ihr Anwendungen, Herausgegeben von Alexander Mitscherlich. *Heft, II*, XXX.

Toulmin, S. (1948). The logical status of psychoanalysis. Reprinted in M. Macdonald (Ed.) *Philosophy and analysis* (pp. 132–138). Oxford: Blackwell, 1954.

Wallerstein, R., & Gill, M. (1991). Letters to the Editors. *Int. Journal Psycho-Analysis, 72*, 159–168.

Weiss, J., & Sampson, H. (1986). *The psychoanalytic process: Theory, clinical observations, and empirical research*. New York: Guilford Press.

Wilkins, W. (1979). Expectations in therapy research: Discriminating among heterogeneous nonspecifics. *Journal of Consulting and Clinical Psychology, 47, 837–845.

Wittgenstein, L. (1922). *Tractatus logico-philosophicus.* London: Kegan Paul.

———. (1953). *Philosophical investigations.* Oxford: Basil Blackwell.

———. (1980). *Culture and value.* G. H. von Wright (Ed.), Peter Winch (trans.). Chicago: University of Chicago Press.

———. (1982). Conversations on Freud: Excerpts from 1932-3 lectures. In R. Wollheim & J. Hopkins (Eds.), *Philosophical essays on Freud* (pp. 1–11). Cambridge: Cambridge University Press.

Wollheim, R., & Hopkins, J. (1982). *Philosophical essays on Freud.* Cambridge: Cambridge University press.

Young-Breuhl, E. (1988). *Anna Freud: A biography.* New York: Summit.

Name Index

A
Abraham, Karl, 53, 67, 77
Adler, A., 134
Alexander, Franz, 63, 131–132
Allport, G. W., 34, 50, 146
Arlow, Jacob, 97, 111, 126, 158

B
Beebe, 21
Bellak, L., 27, 30, 59, 96, 98, 104–105, 130, 137, 148, 151, 158, 162
Bergin, A., 141
Bergman, A., 83, 89
Bernfeld, Siegfried, 76
Bowlby, John, 78–83, 88
Brenner, Charles, 97, 111, 126, 158
Breuer, J., 70

C
Cannon, W., 41
Chassan, J., 151
Chein, I., 30
Ciompi, 151
Clark, R., 72
Compton, Allan, 158

D
Dahl, Hartvig, 151, 152, 153, 160, 161, 162
Drury, M. O'C., 114–115

E
Eissler, K., 37
Erikson, E., 89
Eysenck, Hans, 48, 138–139, 141

F
Federn, 23
Ferenczi, Sandor, 77
Fisher, S., 137
Flew, A., 117, 121
Frank, Jerome, 132
Frank, Philipp, 128
Frege, Gottlieb, 113
Freidlander, B., 92
Freud, Sigmund, 4, 5–6, 41, 42, 53, 56, 58, 60, 61–62, 67, 69–75, 77, 87, 89, 95–96, 97, 114, 116–120, 123, 124, 131, 135, 137, 138, 154–155, 166
Freud, Anna, 75–77, 80, 82, 97
Freud, Sophie, 70
Fries, 16

G

Gadamer, H., G., 121
Gay, P., 72, 73
Gediman, H., 59, 96, 98, 104–105, 151
Gill, Merton, 122, 131
Glass, G., 139
Goldsmith, L., 104
Graf, Herbert, 71–72, 73, 77
Graf, Hermann, 123
Graf, Max, 71
Graf, Rosa, 123
Greenberg, J., 78, 83
Greenberg, R., 137
Greenspan, S., 90–91
Groddeck, G., 61–62
Grosskurth, Phyllis, 76, 80, 82, 83
Grubl, Carl, 123
Grünbaum, Adolf, 126–127

H

Habermas, Jurgen, 121, 122
Halberstadt-Freud, W. Ernst, 70–71, 72–73, 123
Hartmann, Heinz, 57, 58, 97, 125
Heinicke, Christoph, 80
Herbart, C. P., 26
Hersen, M., 137
Holzman, Philip, 36, 122, 135
Hook, Sidney, 111, 124–126, 127–128
Horowitz, Marti, 160, 161, 162
Howard, K., 142
Hurvich, J., 59, 96, 98, 104–105, 151
Huxley, Julian, 80

J

Jacobson, 23, 133
Jones, Ernest, 73, 77, 118
Jung, Carl, 48

K

Kächele, 152, 159, 160, 161
Kant, Immanuel, 115
Kernberg, Otto, 45, 133, 159
Klein, George, 117, 119, 122
Klein, Melanie, 38–39, 45, 59, 75, 77–78, 80, 82, 88
Koch, 134
Koehler, 132
Kopta, S., 142
Krause, M., 142
Kris, Ernst, 6, 155
Kubie, Lawrence, 126

L

Lebovici, Serge, 158
Levin, R., 30
Lichtenberg, 21
"Little Hans," 71–72, 73
Lorenz, Konrad, 80
Luborsky, Lester, 151, 152

M

MacFarlane, J., 92
MacIntyre, A. C., 118, 119–120, 121
Mahler, Gustav, 113
Mahler, Margaret, 45, 83–86, 88, 89, 92
McDougall, William, 50, 59
Michelson, L., 137
Miller, T., 139
Minsky, Marvin, 152
Mitchell, S., 78, 83
Mowrer, O. J., 20, 21
Murphy, G., 30

Murray, Henry, 32–33, 39, 162, 163

N
Nagel, Ernest, 125
Neurath, Otto, 128

O
Orlinsky, D., 142

P
Peterfreund, E., 88–89
Peters, R. S., 117–118, 121
Pine, F., 83, 89
Popper, Karl, 112, 123–124, 126–127, 134
Popper-Lyunkeus, Josef, 123

R
Rapaport, David, 96, 133
Reiff, Philip, 70
Ricoeur, Paul, 121
Riviere, Joan, 78
Robertson, Jimmy, 79
Rogers, Carl, 140
Runes, Dagobert D., 26
Russell, Bertrand, 113

S
Sampson, Harold, 154–156
Sander, 90–91
Sandler, Joseph, 158
Schafer, Roy, 119, 122
Sears, R., 20
Sechehaye, M., 23
Seebohm, T., 121
Shapiro, D., 140
Shapiro, D. A., 140

Sheldon, W., 48, 51
Shevrin, Howard, 159
Smith, M., 139
Spence, Donald, 121, 138, 161
Spitz, Rene, 16, 59, 79, 89, 150
Stern, Dan, 87–94
Stevens, S. S., 2, 145

T
Thomä, 152, 159, 160, 161
Toulmin, S., 116–117, 121

U
Ullman, L., 21

W
Wallerstein, Robert, 131, 158, 159
Weiss, Eduardo, 30
Weiss, Joseph, 151, 153–157
Weisskopf, E. A., 33
Westheimer, Ilse, 80
Wilkins, W., 142
Williams, A., Hyatt, 83
Winnicott, Donald, 45, 82
Wittgenstein, Karl, 112
Wittgenstein, Ludwig, 112–116
Wittgenstein, Margarete, 113
Wittgenstein, Paul, 112–113
Woolf, 16

Y
Young-Breuhl, Elizabeth, 76, 82

Subject Index

A

Adaptive behavior, 34–35
Adaptive regression as ego function, 100, 107
Aggression, 34
Anaclitic object choice, 6–7
Analyzability, predicting, 106–107
Apperception (*see also* Perceptual theory): definition of, 26
Apperceptive distortion, 23, 27–36
Attention Deficit Disorder (ADD), 132–133
Attitudes, 1–14
Audio-recorded psychoanalyses, 20, 159
Autistic perception, 31
Autonomous functioning as ego function, 101, 107

B

Behavioral propositions, 65

C

Case studies, 134, 137–138
Cathexis, 5, 40
Cause/reason criticism (Wittgenstein), 112
Character formation, 15–24
Child analysis, 75–77
Childhood symptomatology, 16
Children's Apperception Test (CAT), 22, 108
Classical psychoanalytical treatment vs. psychoanalytic psychotherapy, 132
Classificatory systems, 48–49
Cognitive projection, 32
Cognitive style, 36
Collateral inferences, 12, 20, 147
Complementary projection, 32–33
Condensation and dreams, 43
Conditioning, 21–24
Controlled experimental research, 157–158
Coping mechanisms, 17, 20–21
Core Conflictual Relationship Theme (CCRT), 152, 153

Core self, 92–93
Correlation coefficients, 150
Crisis intervention, 105–106

D
Defense mechanisms, 21, 40, 41–42
Defensive functioning as ego function, 100, 107
Determinism, 4
Developmental phases (Greenspan), 91
Developmental phases (Sander), 91
Developmental sequence (Mahler), 84–85
Developmental theory, 67–94
  Bowlby, John, 78–83
  current status, 69
  Freud, Anna, 75–77
  Freud, Sigmund, 69–75
  Klein, Melanie, 75, 77–78
  Mahler, Margaret, 83–86
  Stern, Dan, 87–94
Dreams, 22–23, 38, 42–43

E
Ego, 58–61
  characteristics of, 97
  function, 23, 37
    assessment, 9–11
    list of, 99–101
    operational definition, 95–109
      assessing ego functions, 105–109
      Freud, 96–97
      functions, 97–101
      rating ego functions, 101–104

      research project, 104–105
  strength, 40–41
Emergent self, 91–92
Empirical consequences, 155
Externalization, 31–33

F
Falsification criticism (Popper), 112
Figure drawings, 23
Figure-constituents, 33, 39
Figure-ground differentiation, 60
Free association, 44–45, 107
Freud and developmental theory, 69–75
Future of psychoanalysis, 165–166

G
Genetic propositions, 65–66
Gestalt psychology, 162–163
Gestalt theory, 38
Greenspan's developmental phases, 91

H
Hermeneutical perspective, 121
Higher mental functioning, 155

I
Id, 61–62
Imaginative projection, 32
Infant distress, 79
Interrater reliability, 10–11, 105, 148
Interviews, 9
Inverted projection, 27–28

J

Judgment, 23
 as ego function, 99, 106

L

Law of frequency, 20
Law of primacy, 20
Learning theory, 15–24
 oedipus complex, 18–21
 perceptual learning, 21–24
Length of treatment, 142
Leveling, concept of, 36–37
Libidinal development, 51–57
Libido theory, 5, 24, 67–68
 propositions, 68
Logical positivism, 128

M

Mahler's developmental sequence, 84–85
Mastery-competence as ego function, 101, 107
Maternal deprivation, 79–81
Measurement, 2–3, 145
Meta-analysis, 139–140, 142
Metapsychology, 122
 principles, 5–6
Methodology, 1–14
 principles, 3–6
Moral behavior, 62
Mt. Zion project, 153–157

N

Narcissism, 5, 7–8
Nonspecific psychotherapy, 132

O

Object relations theory, 45–46, 133
Object relationship as ego function, 99–100, 107
Object-cathexis, 5, 7–8, 40
Objectivation, 30
Observations as data, 84
Oedipus complex, 18–21, 124
Ordinal scales, 145
Oscillating function of ego, 44
Overdeterminism, 4–5

P

Pathological propositions, 65
Patient's history, 15–16, 146–147
Perception (*see also* Perceptual theory): and clinical phenomena, 40–46
Perceptual learning, 21–24
Perceptual theory, 25–46
Personality, 15–24
 and life history, 134
 oedipus complex, 18–21
 perceptual learning, 21–24
 types, 64–65
Phase specificity, 24
Philosophy and psychoanalysis, 111–128
 bad feelings and suspicion, 111–112
 falsification and standards of science, 124–127
 Popper, Karl, 123–124
 Wittgenstein, Ludwig, 112–116
Postdiction, 12, 20, 146
Predicting analyzability, 106–107
Prediction, 12, 19–20, 146, 149
Principles (*see* Methodology)
Process study, 140

Projection, 23, 27–30
  definition of, 37
Psychoanalysis as form of treatment, 129–164
Psychoanalytic process, definition of, 160
Psychological testing, 108
Psychopharmacology, 106
Psychotherapeutic improvement standards, 139
Psychotropic drugs, study of, 98
Pure perception, 34–36

Q

Quantification, 2

R

Rank ordering, 65–66 (see also Rating scale, ego function; Ratings)
Rating scale, ego function, 9–11
  manual and descriptions, 101–104
Ratings, 84, 156
Reality testing, 23
  as ego function, 99, 106
Recorded sessions, 20
Repressive behavior, 17
Regulation of drives as ego function, 99, 107
Relationship episodes (REs), 152
Repetitive structure ("frames"), 152
Repression, 41
Research:
  in methods, 144–148
  in psychoanalysis, 133–164
    background, 137–143

project, ego function assessment, 104–105
  training, 13
Rorschach test, 35, 108

S

Sander's developmental phases, 91
Schizophrenia research, 158–159
Scientific vs. clinical attitudes, 1–3
Secondary elaboration and dreams, 43
Self, senses of, 91–94
Sense of reality as ego function, 99, 106
Sensitization, 30–31
Separation-individuation, 85
Simple projection, 28–30
Standards of improvement, 139
Stanford-Binet intelligence test, 35
Stimulus barrier as ego function, 100–101, 107
Structural aspects of apperception, 37
Structural theory, 96
Subjective self, 93
Success neurosis, 19
Superego, 62–64
Supplementary projection, 32–33
Symbolization and dreams, 43–44
Synthetic-integration functioning as ego function, 101, 107

T

Tape-recorded sessions, 142
Terminology, 151–152

Thematic Apperception Test (TAT), 21, 27, 32, 33, 34, 35, 108
Third-party payments, 108–109, 166
Thought processes as ego function, 100
Topographic theory, 96
Trait, definition of, 47–48
Trait psychology, 47–66
   ego, 58–61
   id, 61–62
   libidinal development, 51–57
   superego, 62–64
Transcribed sessions, 156
Transcripts of sessions, 148–149, 151
Transference, 130–131, 152
   distortion, 44
   phenomena, 39

V

Verbal self, 93–94
Videotaping, 90, 157